Health Coach Wisdom

YOU HAVE THE POWER TO BE HEALTHY

Lynell Ross

BALBOA.
PRESS

A DIVISION OF HAY HOUSE

Balboa Press books may be ordered through booksellers or by contacting:

Balboa Press
A Division of Hay House
1663 Liberty Drive
Bloomington, IN 47403
www.balboapress.com
1 (877) 407-4847

Cover and interior artwork by Sharon Dean, Creative Accomplice, Inc.

Print information available on the last page.

ISBN: 978-1-5043-3919-3 (sc)
ISBN: 978-1-5043-3920-9 (e)

Library of Congress Control Number: 2015913363

Balboa Press rev. date: 9/16/2015

For my mother Barbara,
who taught me to see the best in others
and to love unconditionally…

Contents

Acknowledgments

With the help of many talented people, I have fulfilled my goal of writing this book. It has been a long journey. Aside from the burning desire I had to shine a light on heart disease and to spread the message that we all have the power to be healthy, what kept me going were the following very special people.

First I want to thank my friend and editor, Debbie Lopez. She a skillful editor, my biggest supporter, has urged me to keep moving forward and to believe in myself. Thank you for being here every step of the way.

A huge thank you to Sharon Dean of Creative Accomplice, Inc. Sharon is a talented graphic designer who created my book cover and many of my interior graphics. She is a true friend who has advised me and lifted my spirits for years. I appreciate your taking your time to work with me even when it seemed like I was never going to finish. Thank you for doing a wonderful job.

Michelle Zuniga of Studio Z Photography is an amazing photographer who has spent many hours shooting photos for my cover and editing my interior photos. Thank you for your hard work and inspiration. You set a high quality standard that I aim to follow.

Carol Riggs is a compassionate and wise teacher and life coach who inspired me to write my first cookbook over a decade ago. Carol not only introduced me to coaching and gave me the courage to do what I love; she pointed me in a direction that completely changed my life. Your guidance has made me a better parent, friend and a more peaceful person.

Erik Olesen not only wrote the foreword for my book, but he helped me navigate the rough waters of self-awareness. Thank you Erik for being a wise mentor and for helping me to build my confidence, become a more compassionate communicator and for giving me the tools to move from fear to love.

Patricia Carpizo Kauffman is an angel that teaches more than just yoga and meditation. She teaches the union of mind and body, how to open your heart and be grateful. Thank you my friend for teaching me all that and showing me how to slow down and appreciate each moment of this glorious life. Thank you for demonstrating yoga and exercise poses for my fitness chapter.

Thank you to my friends and family who allowed us to capture your photos while living your own healthy lifestyle so that I may share your enthusiasm for life and inspire others to do the same. Thank you to my husband John, my sons Matt and John, his wife, Alaina, and to my extended family for your support during this project and for showing me what true love is. Thank you to Renee Meade, Patricia Kauffman and Mariscela Alvarez for gracing the cover with your beautiful smiles and for your inspiring stories.

Thank you Ashlie Pechin, of FitForce Bootcamp, for demonstrating exercises, for your encouragement, and for helping me to take my fitness to the next level.

Thank you to Marcos Maykall and Professor Clare Dendinger for teaching me how to prepare healthy, yet delicious meals by cutting back on sugar, salt and fat while replacing them with enthusiasm and love. Thank you also to Debbie Lucus and Janet Moore, my encouraging Registered Dietician friends who helped me make peace with food and for showing me how to share my message with your bright, positive, funny and easy going teaching styles.

Thank you to Therese Pope for your initial editing and encouragement to add my own story. Thank you to Brooke Higgins for your guidance on communicating my message in a more direct way. Your advice has been invaluable.

I send my gratitude to my first boss, Tom Liguori who installed confidence in me at a young age by believing in me then, and now by encouraging me to complete this book. How fortunate I was to be guided by a leader who treated me with respect and compassion and allowed me to try my own ideas. Thank you also for teaching me about Action Plans. I have used them in every area of my life.

Thank you to José and Barbara Kirchner for your support, for bringing me authentic cookbooks from all over the Mediterranean and for mentoring me to be a better speaker and instructor.

Another angel in my life has been Ingrid Goff-Maidoff, writer and poet. She has inspired me to be a kinder person and encouraged me to coach happiness, the ultimate source of well-being. She is the definition of grace.

I would be lost without my circle of friends, Margaret Slane, Diana Arndt, Sandi Thys, Renee Meade, Sandy Amara, Phyllis Classon, Susan Rhodes, Stephanie Watson, Becky Thurmon, Valerie Godsey, Laurie Smith, Carol French and Debbie Lopez. I have learned about healthy and better living from these wise women. They have shared recipes and health tips, helped me with my computer and technology, sampled my recipe creations, let me drag them on hikes, sat through my workshops and have encouraged me in every way. Most of all they set the gold standard for what it means to be true friends.

I am truly blessed with what I call my "Dream Team" of friends and a wonderful family. My husband, sons, sisters, cousins, brothers and sisters in-law, nieces and nephews have been the inspiration behind my desire to learn about wellness. I especially appreciate the support from my husband John, no matter what path I have taken. Being encouraged by my sister Michelle made a difference when I felt afraid. I want to thank my family for believing in me.

In addition, I created a *virtual dream team* of mentors and teachers that have helped me to create a better life. As I began to develop a healthy lifestyle, I turned to experts who were examples of the kind of person I wanted to be. I want to thank the following leaders for their work and for guiding us all to be healthier, happier and for encouraging us to be our best by stepping out and doing great things for the world.

Thank you to Dr. Wayne Dyer for your teachings. From you I learned to overcome self-defeating thoughts and to be courageous enough to follow my heart and live my purpose. Thank you to Cheryl Richardson for being gracious enough to answer my questions on your radio show and in your workshops. I have followed the advice in your books, doing everything from building up my coaching practice, to setting boundaries to creating an *exceptional life*. I use too many of your tools and insights to mention here, and my favorite is your brilliant idea that keeps me moving forward, your "Absolute Yes List." I write a new list of my top five priorities each season, and thanks to you I focus on my values and goals, which allows me to sort out distractions. What a great teacher and gift you have been to me.

From Michael Neill I learned that nothing is impossible. Thank you for your insight in helping me to believe I could finish this book. From Dr. Robert Holden I learned about forgiveness, and how easy it is to be truly happy by connecting with my higher self. From Alan Cohen I discovered true peace of mind. From Louise Hay I learned that our thoughts create our reality and our health. I would like to thank Louise Hay for being a shining example of how to appreciate each moment and how to be more kind and loving to ourselves and to each other. Thank you all for making our world a better place.

Foreword

Several years ago, I spent two weeks traveling in Brazil, capped by four days in beautiful Rio de Janeiro. One day, on my way to the famed beach at Copacabana, I watched a family walking along the sidewalk. It was a sun swept day, with a temperature of 80 degrees, and a light breeze. The family - a mother, father, and two small children, appeared to be quite poor. Yet as they walked, with the light blue ocean of the Bay before them, they laughed and played with each other. Watching them, relaxed and happy with each other, I felt myself relaxing too. I will never forget that moment, and the joy, love, and immersion in the present moment the small family showed.

After flying back to the United States, we caught a shuttle back to where the car was parked. Watching the other vehicles around me, I saw tension and seriousness in the eyes and movements of the drivers. Through this was the San Francisco Bay Area, affluent and trendy, the people driving those cars did not look happy. I thought fondly of that family in Rio, remembering how relaxed and happy they looked, though they obviously had much less money than any of those driving around me. I felt sad, thinking of what many people have traded for a "higher" standard of living.

What, then, is the difference between that happy family and the tense drivers I saw near San Francisco? Both lived in a world renowned city. Both had access to a beautiful, natural environment. Yet the family in Rio, in spite of much less money, seemed much more happy.

In the book you are about to read, Health Coach Lynell Ross does not directly address the differences above. Yet she focused on what underlies them - the choices that we make in our lives - choices that lead to health, wellness, and happiness. We, in the "First World" have amazing access to technology, entertainment, and resources. Yet, often, through our choices, we end up having significantly less contentment and health than we might otherwise. In a masterful way, Lynell helps us to understand why. More important, this book provides the tools to help us change the lifestyle choices we make. Lynell calls these essential tools "Secrets", and in this book, she teaches us how to unlock them. And indeed, five of the secrets were exhibited by the family at Copacabana Beach.

I've known Lynell Ross for a number of years. Lynell is unique - a superbly trained Health Coach, with many years of experience in her field. She is certified by the foremost group for training and recognizing Health Coaches through the Wellcoaches School of Coaching. The process she went through to gain this certification was rigorous and in depth. Yet her experience isn't what's most impressive about Lynell. What's amazing is her commitment, focus, and determination.

Whenever I meet with Lynell, she shows up with notes about what she's working on - both professionally and personally. She's always excited to talk about what she's learned about herself and the world. Many coaches and therapists are focused on changing others. They forget to take care of themselves and their own growth. This is where Lynell is different than most health professionals and coaches. She knows that practicing the Secrets for herself will help her to help others.

So, what are these Secrets? In this book, Lynell covers eight:

- Your Thoughts Create Your Life
- The Healing Power of Nutrition
- Fitting Fitness Into Your Daily Routine
- Be Socially Connected in a Healthy Way
- Reduce Stress and Live a Joyful Life
- Where Personal Growth Meets Spirituality
- Find Peace with your Sense of Purpose
- Sleeping Well and Other Wellness Strategies

In this book you will learn to apply these Health Coach Secrets to transform your life. In addition, she includes great recipes, all approved by nutritionists, that will help you transform your table, and your body. And Lynell doesn't take a "fad" approach to nutrition. She recommends approaches that can be tailored to help anyone.

Lynell writes that 80-90% of disease is preventable, and I agree. It reminds me of an oft quoted statistic that is equally valid - 90% of all disease is stress related. When I taught Biofeedback and Neurofeedback at San Francisco State University, we helped students learn how they could change the way their bodies worked - hand temperature, muscular tension, and even the electrical activity of the brain. The upshot of all this? By making the right choices, and learning important strategies, we have great power to change our lives and to remain healthy. And if you are reading this book because you are dealing with a health challenge, Lynell will show you how these same lifestyle choices will help you regain vibrant health.

Most of us don't live in a tropical paradise, like Rio de Janeiro. Yet we can learn to make choices and live our lives to regain health and happiness, even when we're struggling with stress and other challenges. In this important book, Lynell Ross shows us exactly how to do it.

Erik Olesen, MS, MFT
Licensed Psychotherapist (California), Corporate Consultant
BCIA Certified Biofeedback and Neurofeedback Trainer
Author of *Mastering the Winds of Change: Peak Performers Reveal How to Stay on Top in Times of Turmoil*, Erik lives in Auburn, California.

Introduction

Regardless of how you feel right now, as you begin to practice the strategies in this book, you will change your health and life for the better. I know it is possible because I have not only learned the secrets of becoming healthy and fit, I have practiced them. I had a compelling reason to learn about health. Most all of my family, including my mother, grandparents, cousins, aunts and uncles, have been affected by or died prematurely from heart disease. The frustration I felt from watching people I loved suffer, without knowing how to take care of their health, motivated me to learn how to eat and live well. I felt an urgent need to help others prevent the pain of stroke, heart attack and missing out on their life. The key to feeling great, maintaining a healthy weight and being happy is by focusing on wellness and listening to your own needs.

When you are finished reading and taking the action steps in *Health Coach Wisdom*, you will have more energy, be less stressed, and know how to create the healthy and happy life you deserve. It is easier than you have been told to feel great, have good relationships, enjoy peace of mind, lose weight and keep it off—*for good*. The answer lies in caring about yourself and understanding your motivations. You'll learn about the power of nutrition and its affect on your life. I've studied in the fields of nutrition, fitness and positive psychology to find these answers. I learned how to cook healthy foods that make life pleasurable. The recipes in *Health Coach Wisdom* have been approved and edited by a Registered Dietitian. In addition, many of my recipes were approved by Registered Dietitians when used in teaching the Diabetes Prevention Program at our local health clinic. The participants were happy to learn how delicious fresh and healthy foods taste.

Every choice you make either puts you on the path to good health or poor health. Focus your attention on developing a healthy lifestyle and you will create a naturally fit body and a peaceful mind.

The Biggest Secret of All is Hidden Within You

You hold the key to your own health and happiness. *Believe* that you deserve to be healthy and happy. You are perfect as you are right now, a good, kind and loving person. Mistakes you have made are in the past and are not "failures"; they are lessons on your life's path.

Resolve to be a person who treats yourself well and inspires others. Learn the basic facts about the components of a healthy lifestyle while you listen to your own inner wisdom. In *Health Coach Wisdom* you will discover...

8 Steps to Your Healthy Weight and Vibrant Life

Step 1: Your Thoughts Create Your Health. It is your thoughts and beliefs that hold you back from living your healthiest life. The way to create lasting health is to start from the inside, to change the way you think about your health. We will make a plan to focus on your health, and then we will examine what is most important to you.

Step 2: Eat Well: The Healing Power of Nutrition. Anyone can eat well. It doesn't matter if you are single, married, work full time, have a family, or don't have a lot of money. Eating is very personal, yet there are some nutritional benefits that most experts agree upon. Nourish yourself with powerful nutrients eaten in proper portions for your needs to reach your healthy weight. You will find answers to your eating dilemmas, delicious healthy recipes and meal planning ideas to keep you motivated.

Step 3: Weave Fitness into Your Daily Routine. Think it can't be done? Maybe you don't know how easy it can be to weave fitness in throughout your day. You will discover that being fit and keeping your heart healthy is easier than you think. You'll find tips that show you how to become strong, fit and healthy, one day at a time.

Step 4: Be Socially Connected in a Healthy Way. One of the key components to health is being socially connected with good relationships. "Social networking" has taken on a whole new meaning. Stay connected to others in a real and meaningful way, and not just through the computer. We must be careful not to disconnect from important people in our daily lives. Learn the secrets to building strong and healthy relationships.

Step 5: Reduce Stress and Live a Joyful Life. We can choose how we perceive the events in our lives. Learn how to reduce and even eliminate stress so that we are able to accept the life we deserve. Fun is one of the most overlooked steps in creating a joyful, healthy life. Have fun each day. You deserve it and your health depends on it.

Step 6: Where Personal Growth Meets Spirituality. The doorway to vitality opens by growing and continually learning something new. If you don't water and nurture your garden, not even the weeds will grow. When you slow down and become quiet, you deepen your spiritual connection by hearing your inner voice of true wisdom. You will gain strength, vision and a new appreciation for life's lessons. Being your best self not only inspires others, it will improve our world.

Step 7: Find Peace with Your Sense of Purpose. Purpose means something different to everyone. The main theme of this book is: *You have the power.* On some level, you know your purpose but may have not fully tapped into it yet. In this step we examine ways for you to find meaning and purpose in your life.

Step 8: Sleep and Other Wellness Strategies. Lack of sleep can be hazardous to your health and create a cascade of problems. Neglecting things like dental care and other necessary health routines directly affect our ability to thrive. Learn how to take proactive steps to safeguard your health and prevent illness by creating healthy habits.

You can create a healthy lifestyle without spending a lot of money, time, or even making big changes. Healthy habits are very simple. I have spent years discovering health secrets from people who are thriving and living vibrant lives. From this knowledge I share 8 steps to health and happiness. In each chapter you will find tips that I call "Health Coach Wisdom." These are key ideas that I have gathered through working with clients, experts and my own lessons learned. Throughout the book you will find circle bullet points, numbered lists and heart shaped bullet points. I designed this book to be easy to read, and to provide you with quick reference lists. The heart shaped bullets represent ideas to try or helpful information for the heart. The other bullets provide interesting facts and the numbers provide you with steps to take.

Much of this book is filled with health information, woven with stories from my experience with friends, family and clients. If you really want to make a shift to improve your health and happiness, then the driving force behind this plan is you. You get to choose what is best for you, by connecting with your mind, body and spirit. Each area of your life is connected to the other, so when you make balanced choices; you create your vision of health and happiness. Let's start your wellness journey and help you discover what you've known all along—*you have the power to be healthy!*

Lynell Ross

Chapter 1

Your Thoughts Determine Your Health

You have been given the greatest power in the world, the power to choose.
~Denis Waitley

♥ **Health Coach Wisdom:** Our mental attitude determines the quality of our health.

"I know what to do, so why don't I do it?"Almost everyone I talk to about health and fitness asks me this. In order to be a good health coach, I needed to find the answers. After years of research and working with people, I have uncovered many reasons why people don't take better care of their health. Can you find any that apply to you?

- ♥ We make being healthy and fit more complicated than it is.
- ♥ We *think* staying fit and losing weight is more difficult than it is because we do not understand the basic facts about nutrition and fitness.
- ♥ We are blocked by past events that prevent us from moving forward.
- ♥ We operate most of the time from sub-conscious habits.
- ♥ We are stuck in our beliefs, which may or may not be true.
- ♥ We are angry or disappointed with ourselves and have given up.
- ♥ We forget to make health a priority.
- ♥ We get distracted and are not aware of our actions. We are not being mindful.
- ♥ We don't know what we want or don't believe it is possible.
- ♥ We don't have a plan.
- ♥ We have not uncovered our own motives for change.
- ♥ We don't listen to our own inner wisdom.

These are compelling reasons for not changing, yet by harnessing the power of your mind, you can change your health for the better, and it is much easier than you think. If more people understood the basics of nutrition, the benefits of being physically fit, and how to reduce stress, we may not have the health or obesity crisis that we have in our country today. Most people confuse being healthy with what they weigh, yet a person's *weight is only one part of good health.* There are several components to wellness that together create a whole healthy and happy life.

Creating a Healthy Lifestyle Is the Key to Wellness

Whatever the mind can conceive and believe, it can achieve.
~Napoleon Hill

What do you believe about your health and your future? Many of us don't take time to think about creating a healthy lifestyle because we don't believe we can. We suppress our feelings and often live with anxiety. Many people either accept being overweight or spend their lives going on and off diets. Those who create healthy lifestyles are physically fit and maintain a healthy weight without dieting. A primary step in developing a healthy lifestyle is to learn how to transform *negative* thoughts and feelings into *positive* ones.

It is not only possible to feel good, it is possible to thrive fully when you bring the power of your mind together your physical body and listen to your spirit. Believe, without a doubt, you have the power to heal and live the life you dream about.

How? It is not difficult. It is a journey, an adventure. When focusing on the components of wellness, you are giving yourself a gift. Think of each day as an opportunity to be kind to yourself while choosing what you need for optimal health. Each chapter of this book focuses on a key area of wellness. You can take action to propel yourself to the next level of living well by discovering the following:

1. Your **thoughts and beliefs** direct your level of health.
2. The **foods you eat** can heal your body and mind.
3. Being **fit and flexible** can prevent pain and injury.
4. Your **social connections and healthy relationships** support your well-being.
5. Your **life's purpose and meaning are** what keep you going.
6. You can live a **joy**-filled life with little or no stress.
7. Your personal growth and your **spirituality** lead to vitality.
8. Reducing risky behaviors and learning **to sleep well** support the quality of your health and life.

After being aware of our thoughts, the next step in improving our mental outlook is **through good nutrition** and **exercise,** which helps us manage stress. Having a positive outlook involves more than just trying to snap out of a bad mood. This book will provide you with resources for transforming negative thoughts and behaviors to help you set yourself up for health success.

In making your health a priority, you will begin to feel better right away. Your body will begin to heal, and your mind will become clear. You will make better choices and think more rationally. You will be calm and better able to handle stressors. By putting your health and well-being at the top of your list, everything else will fall into place. Your relationships will improve, you will perform better at work and have the confidence to grow and change. Great health equals a great life!

> Your life changes the moment you make a new, congruent
> and committed decision. ~ Tony Robbins

Our Lives Are Shaped by Our Thoughts

From the time we are young children, we are judged by peers, parents, teachers, coaches, and family. These sometimes-critical judgments can leave scars on our hearts and in our minds. We may grow up thinking we are not enough. Critical messages run through our heads like the news stream at the bottom of a television screen. We strive to do better, yet often it feels overwhelming and we give up. You have the ability to think differently.

Once you make the decision to improve your health, you may feel overwhelmed and might need the help of a coach, support group, or books to help you begin thinking in a new way. Books are great tools for change, as are affirmations, *positive statements that we repeat to ourselves.* Such support is helpful because we often carry guilt, and it is difficult to shift our thinking alone. To move forward, we need to forgive ourselves and others for past mistakes. Guilt and shame serve no purpose unless we use the truth to learn from our mistakes and move forward.

We need to believe that we deserve to be healthy and happy. It takes patience to learn to love and care for ourselves. What you *believe* about what you eat and about exercise and stress determines how you feel and how you behave. If you walk for twenty minutes and tell yourself that isn't good enough, you will drain your energy. If you eat something you enjoy and tell yourself you "shouldn't have," you create stress. Learn to support yourself by making good choices *and affirming them.*

♥ **Health Coach Wisdom:** Use affirmations to boost your self-confidence and change your outlook. Write positive affirmations on three-by-five cards, and post them where you will see them every day.

Affirmations are statements you make that create your life. If you are careful about your thoughts, you can create the health you want. Good health comes from the day-in and day-out healthy habits that you practice on a consistent basis. Read these affirmations to create healthy habits, or choose your own, write them down, and post them where you see them throughout your day.

- I enjoy making healthy habits fun and I laugh every day.
- I create a healthy body and mind by being kind to myself.
- I meet my friends to walk and talk instead of sitting.
- I eat five to eleven servings of fruits and vegetables daily.
- My car is cell free. I do not text or talk on the cell phone while driving.
- I always wear my seat belt.
- I speak in positives. I do not complain.

Every thought I think and every word I speak is an affirmation for my future.
~ Louise L. Hay

Focus on Your Health, and You Will Be Rewarded Every Day.

When you feel good, you can do almost anything. You can face problems and enjoy your life. When you are ill or in pain, even the simplest of tasks can seem impossible. If your number-one priority is being well you will make a habit of doing healthy things that make you feel good. You can prevent illness and injury by practicing simple healthy habits.

With good health and a good attitude, all things are possible. Do you set yourself up for success when it comes to your health? Do you think of your foods and beverages as providing you with the nutrition your body needs? Do you make the connection that moving your body is strengthening your bones and muscles to avoid injury? Do you take the time you need for rest and relaxation?

The key to being well lies in building good health habits into your everyday life, *not waiting until another time.* But how do you get started?

Begin with the End Goal

Start with the end in mind
~ Stephen R. Covey, *7 Habits of Highly Effective People*

Many people wait until a crisis happens before they take action. You can avoid disaster by being clear about what you want. Begin with the end goal in mind. If your goal is to be healthy, to reach a healthy weight, or to be more physically fit, then focus on that goal *now*. In this chapter, you will find a simple tool for creating a plan that works for you. When you feel overwhelmed, how do you gain control of your life so you can focus on your goal? One of your problems may be that you are using your energy worrying about other people and creating drama instead of focusing on your own needs. Dr. Henry Cloud, in his book, *The One-Life Solution* offers the following advice for gaining control of our time:

> ...most people are so caught up in trying to control the things they cannot control—other people, circumstances, or outcomes, that in the process they lose control of themselves. And here is the real paradox. It is only when you do take control of yourself that you will begin to have significant influence on those other people and circumstances.

The Law of Power

All loss of power comes from you, not from other people. The reason is that power over yourself is all you ever had anyhow, so it is the only kind of power that you can ever gain or lose. You have the power to control yourself and nothing else, including other people. When you understand that, then you begin to truly get in control of yourself and your life while letting others be who they are.

The Secret to a Healthy Life: Clear Vision

When you change the way you look at things, the things you look at change.
~Wayne Dyer, *Change Your Thoughts-Change Your Life*

Sit quietly and look into your future. When it comes to your health, there are two paths you can take, each resulting in a very different outcome.

Path One: In following the first path, one that many Americans are on, you go through your daily life not thinking about what you eat and drink. You often relieve stress with food, alcohol, shopping or surfing the internet. You don't take action toward becoming physically fit. You tell yourself you are too tired to move.

Path Two: In following the other path, you take time to think about the health you want. You consider the things and people most important to you. You prioritize your values. You organize your time, plan your meals and are active throughout your day. You spend your time on things that help you mentally and physically.

Consider the Outcomes

Path One: By believing that *little things* don't matter, you wake up one day to find that you are out of shape and not physically fit. Here are the consequences:

- This is how most back pain and injuries start. Your muscles, ligaments and tendons may be weak. You pick up a heavy box and immediately injure yourself. This can be a dangerous and painful journey, a slippery slope to being out of work, taking pain killers, or facing surgery.
- You may go to the doctor with knee pain and learn that you need surgery, but they won't perform the knee surgery until you lose weight because the extra pounds you are carrying will continue to cause you problems.
- You don't feel well and your doctor informs you that you are pre-diabetic and if you do not lose weight and become more active, you will need medication. At your next visit you are told that you need medication to control your blood sugar and your dangerously-high blood pressure. You now have type 2 diabetes.
- You may have a heart attack or stroke and are lucky enough to survive, but now you face a long and slow recovery. Your whole life changes; you have lost your freedom, your mobility and your health.

Path Two: By building healthy lifestyle habits, you create total well-being:

- You wake up every morning feeling great. You choose healthy foods daily.
- Even if you feel a little stiff you take part in a regular fitness routine such as stretching, yoga, or walking *and you immediately feel better.*
- You keep your cardiovascular system healthy by walking, jogging, swimming or biking. You enjoy a well rounded life, play golf, go hiking, skiing, kayaking or participate in exercise classes.
- You enjoy your work because you feel good all the time, full of energy and humor. You work in your garden, volunteer, ride bikes, play sports and take up new hobbies with new friends.

♥ You travel often and very rarely get sick. You don't get headaches, sinus infections or suffer from a bad back. You are strong, physically fit and have a great attitude about life.

Prepare for a Healthy Lifestyle Change

Be resolved and the thing is done.

~Confucius

Before planning to change a behavior, it is helpful to understand the steps for successful behavior modification. Whether you wish to lose weight, become physically fit, eat better, stop smoking, or exercise more, the process to change is the same. Ask yourself questions such as: How long do I want to live? What quality of life do I want to have?

People who believe they have control over their lives have an internal locus of control, while people with an external locus of control believe what happens to them is a result of chance and is unrelated to their behavior. Most people fall somewhere in the middle. They *fail to see the connection between their choices and how each one affects their health.* To understand your motivations, let's examine the **stages of change:**

1. **Pre-contemplation** (*You are not even thinking about it*)
2. **Contemplation** (*You begin to consider change*)
3. **Preparation** (*You start making a plan*)
4. **Action** (*You make changes for 6 months*)
5. **Termination/Adoption** (*You successfully change for 5 years*)
6. **Maintenance** (*The new change becomes a lifelong habit*)

Think of one thing you might want to change. Where are you on this scale regarding your plans to take action? Before you begin your steps to change, be aware of the **barriers to change:**

1. We **procrastinate** (We *think it will be easier to start tomorrow*)
2. We have **pre-conditioned beliefs** (*About weight loss and health*)
3. We **want instant gratification** (*We do not want to wait to be healthy and fit*)
4. We think it is too **complicated** (*To learn about health and nutrition*)
5. We **feel helpless** or we don't care anymore (*We give up*)
6. We **rationalize** our bad behaviors (*One more drink won't hurt*)
7. We have illusions of **invincibility** (*We don't think about the long-term effects*)

If you can relate to any of these thoughts, then the most powerful thing you can do for yourself is to resolve to take better care of yourself *today.* Be realistic about your health goals, starting with small changes. Realize that it will take time to reach your goals, yet, *you can enjoy* the journey. Be truthful about the changes you need to make and focus on making the journey easy and fun. If you make a poor choice, then make a better one next time, but do not give up.

Focus on Solutions

When you are open to new ways of thinking, you can always find a solution to a problem. You may not like the answer or the outcome may not be what you had originally planned, but if you really want to achieve your health goal, you will do whatever it takes to reach your destination. Here is a key: *You don't have to try so hard.* Just start thinking about a vision of your healthy self and make choices with that vision in mind. You never fail unless you give up permanently. If you learn something from a mistake, it becomes a lesson, not a failure.

The power **to be** who you want to be, **do what** you want to do and **have what** you want to have comes from within you. When you focus on good health, you feel better. As you feel better you will be able to do things that you love and that matter to you. Our bodies are designed to be well. We become ill when we hurt ourselves by overeating, drinking too much, not exercising or exercising improperly and not sleeping enough.

What is your Wellness Vision?

Take a few minutes to think about and write down your vision below or get a spiral notebook or journal for the exercises in this book. *It is proven that writing down your goals and intentions makes success much more likely.*

Answer these questions or fill in your own wellness vision in a journal:

1. What does a healthy lifestyle look like for you? Who are you with?
2. How do you feel? How would you like to feel?
3. What do you do every day to support your self-care?
4. If you were healthy and fit, what other goals and dreams would you like to accomplish?
5. What would you like your health to look like in one month, six months, one year and five years?
6. Do you have specific health concerns right now? What will happen if you don't take action regarding these concerns?

7. My wellness vision is that I am: _____
   _____
   _____
   _____.

You Have the Power to Be Healthy at Every Age

The secret of getting ahead is getting started.
The secret of getting started is breaking your complex overwhelming tasks
into small manageable tasks and then starting on the first one.
~Mark Twain

People often feel hopeless because of the choices they have made. They turn away from what they need to face and they give up because making changes seems too hard. If you shift your attitude from self-defeating thoughts to self-empowering ones you can begin to make changes **one step at a time**. Great things come from a sequence of small things. You will begin to feel better the instant you decide to make positive changes. *You are what you think you are.* You know what is best for you. Having good health is simple if you go back to basics.

5 Proven Steps to Achieving Your Goals

Faith is substance;
It is the powerful ability to believe in something you cannot see.
~ Jim Rhon

1. **IMAGINE** your goal. Visualize yourself living the life you were meant to live, feeling great, free, light, energetic and wonderful.
2. **BELIEVE** it is possible. If you don't believe you can do it, you won't be able to make *it* happen. *Be your own best friend, value yourself and be your own health coach.*
3. **TAKE ACTION** with a plan. Create your *Action Plan* when you want to achieve anything. Remembering your goal will pull you through. (*See the example later in this chapter.*) When you know why you want to achieve your goal, your plan and reason will prevent you from giving up.
4. **ESTABLISH SUPPORT**. When you try to accomplish something new, it is important to have someone *you can trust* to turn to when you reach difficult time. This can be a friend, a partner or a coach. Make sure this person supports *your* goal and has your best interest at heart.

5. **FOLLOW THROUGH**. This is the last and most critical piece of the puzzle. Many times people start off on a new goal with good intentions and stick with it for a while, and then something happens to take their attention off their goal, and they forget about it. Most people give up just before they are about to have their breakthrough. Establish strategies and reminders to keep you going. Never give up.

♥ **Health Coach Wisdom:** Transform your inner critic into your inner health coach!

How to Determine Your Core Values to Make Better Choices

My dear friend Carol Riggs is an amazing teacher and Life Coach. For years she has been helping me make changes and grow into a more kind and conscious person. The first thing Carol did when we began working together was to help me to determine my core values and what was most important to me. She helped me pinpoint the areas where I was overwhelmed and felt drained and out of control. In order to make positive changes, Carol worked with me to set goals and let go of things that drain my energy. Carol shared her solution for helping me clarify my values and priorities. She asked me to look at the key areas of my life: Health, Finances, Personal Development, Fun & Recreation, Career, Friends and Family, Environment, Significant Other.

She pointed out that each area of our life affects the other. Many people get so caught up in their daily routine that they are unable to step back and see where changes need to be made. Working with Carol as my life coach has been invaluable to me. She has helped me recognize and appreciate what is most important in my life, freeing me up to accomplish more than I had dreamed of. Because I was able to see clearly, I was able to slow down and spend more time on things that mattered most such as making nutritious meals for my family and taking time out to enjoy being with them. In essence, I was creating a healthy lifestyle for my whole family.

After working with Carol's "Key Areas of Life" and studying in the field of nutrition and fitness, I was inspired to create my HEALTH WHEEL DIAGRAM. Review the "Health Wheel" worksheet. Each area is critical to your health. If even one part is out of balance, your health can suffer. If you feel overwhelmed, you are likely to put off paying attention to your health, unless you have very strong healthy habits.

How to Use Your Wheel of Health to Develop a Healthy Lifestyle

♥ **Health Coach Wisdom:** Fill out the Health Wheel. When you are done, review to see if you have a large well-balanced wheel or if unbalanced, which areas can you begin to improve?

Health & Harmony Wellness Coaching

YOUR HEALTH WHEEL
How balanced is your health?

Directions: The outer edge is a 10, and the inner point is a 0. Rank your place in each health area by drawing a dot representing the number each area represents for you. Draw a curved circle by connecting the dots to create a new outer edge. How balanced is your health?

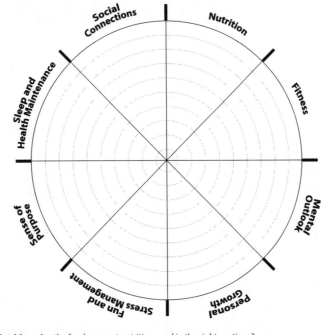

Nutrition: Are the foods you eat nutritious and in the right portions?

Exercise: Do you move throughout the day getting 30 minutes of physical activity?

Social Network: Do you have close friends, family, co-workers, church groups?

Mental Outlook: Do you manage your stress and have a positive attitude?

Sense of Purpose: Do you have a passion? Do you volunteer, help others, teach?

Fun & Stress Management: Do you take time for play? Cope with stress?

Sleep & Health Maintenance: Do you get 7-8 hours of sleep? Take risks?

Personal Growth: Do you continually learn new things & keep current?

Created by Lynell Ross- Health & Harmony Wellness Coaching©

Think Big and Think Small

It is a paradoxical principle of life that the most likely way to reach a goal is to be aiming not at the goal itself but at some more ambitious goal beyond it.
~ Arnold Toynbee

A big factor in helping you build a lifestyle of healthy habits is to have a thrilling goal, something that excites you and a compelling vision for your life. If you have a secret dream of taking a special vacation, starting your own business, solving a problem that will help the planet or being healthy enough to enjoy your family and friends, then taking action toward your dreams will awaken a burning motivation in you. Excitement will propel you to achieve your big goals, allowing you to follow through effortlessly on simple healthy habits, *because you have reasons to be healthy.*

The Formula for Achieving Your Goals

The proven method for achieving your goal is to make it **SMART:**

Specific—**M**easurable—**A**ttainable—**R**easonable **T**ime-bound

Here are a few examples of SMART goals:
- I am eating at least one fruit and vegetable with each meal.
- I will begin my exercise program by walking 10 minutes, three times per week. After week two, I will walk for 20 minutes per day. At week three, I will walk for 30 minutes, 5 days per week.
- I go to bed by 10pm on weeknights to get a good night's sleep.
- I drink 8 eight-ounce cups of water every day.

Most people don't achieve their goals because they make them too big and unrealistic with no time frame, and because they do not have a plan of action. *For example, a key to successful weight loss is to focus on something other than losing weight as your primary goal.* You can achieve your ideal weight naturally by creating a vision of how you want to feel, and how you see yourself in the future.

For each area on your wheel, use an Action Plan—a very powerful tool that will help you focus on achieving your desired goal. Here is how it works: List the steps it takes to complete your project or goal. You will be amazed at how successful you will be by using this technique. It is proven that you are much more likely to achieve a goal **when you**

write it down. Goals can seem far away, but when you break it down into small steps you easily chip away at them. *Taking action prevents you from feeling frustrated or getting stuck and helps you to feel better about yourself.*

♥ **Health Coach Wisdom:** Keep your Action Plan where you will see it.

ACTION PLAN

Project/Goal/Intention: _____

| <u>Action Steps</u> | <u>Due Date</u> |

o _____
o _____
o _____
o _____
o _____
o _____
o _____
o _____
o _____
o _____
o _____
o _____

How to Create a Healthy Lifestyle

What does it mean to create a healthy lifestyle? It means to make healthy choices most of the time. Use the 80/20 rule. Make healthy choices as often as possible on a daily basis, and when you want to treat yourself or relax, do so without feeling guilty *because you trust yourself to make good choices.* In order to want to make a healthy choice instead of an unhealthy choice, you need to:

1. **Understand why you are making the healthy choice**
2. **Be prepared to make a better choice**

Studies show that without prior planning or education, your brain will choose immediate gratification over reason. In other words, when tempted by the aroma of a cinnamon roll as you walk through the airport, you are likely to stop and give in *if you have not pre-programmed yourself to know better.* We live our lives based on habits, surviving on auto pilot, unconsciously moving through our day. Creating a healthy lifestyle means building on healthy habits, one at a time. Research shows that focusing on a new habit for twenty-eight days is sufficient time to make it a permanent habit. What if you took twelve healthy habits and worked on one each month for a whole year? Imagine the changes you could make! If you are thinking, "I don't want to wait a whole year to see changes", then consider this: At the end of this year, you will either, be in the same shape you are now, worse shape or by making small changes, once choice at a time, you can start feeling better right now and have the health you want, permanently. You will build life-long healthy habits.

How do you create a new habit?

You create a new habit by consciously deciding to do something. The key is to reinforce that new behavior with reminders, with a support person, a group meeting, a journal and or tracking system. It takes 28 days to make a new habit stick. Another way to stop a bad habit is to replace it with a good habit. The term for this is called "countering" or replacing one behavior with another. For example, if you want to quit drinking soda, one way to support yourself is to replace your soda with sparkling water and fruit slices over crushed ice.

You Can Create the Healthy Lifestyle *You Want*

We could all use a little coaching.
When you're playing the game, it's hard to think of everything.
~ Jim Rhon

♥ **Health Coach Wisdom:** Make healthy habits a part of your everyday life. Forget "dieting" to lose weight and concentrate on being healthy and feeling great! Create your very own healthy lifestyle.

Winning Strategies to Create Healthy Habits

There is a reason that you picked up this book and started to read it. Maybe you received a bad diagnosis from your doctor, you developed type 2 diabetes, arthritis, suffered a heart attack, stroke, or are unhappy with your weight or lack of physical fitness. If you want to learn an easier way to live a healthy lifestyle, you will find your answers here. This book is about living life on YOUR terms and making choices that work for YOU. It is easy to develop healthy habits when you use strategies developed from experts in the field of health and wellness combined with coaching tips to help you make your own lifelong healthy lifestyle plan.

Creating a Healthy Lifestyle: An Easy Solution to a Big Problem

I began my journey to find out what I should be eating after I was told that I had "high cholesterol— it was 297 when I was only 25 years old. I struggled with what to eat and had no idea what fitness or nutrition was. Back then I had no idea that there was a link to losing both of my grandfathers and grandmothers, a deadly mistake that would cost me the life of my mother. I realized the answers too late to help her. My journey started with learning about nutrition and came full circle when I finally discovered how to prevent heart disease and type 2 diabetes, discovering what it means to live a healthy lifestyle. I have found, through years of research, that the things we need to do for our health are very simple.

I have spent years studying the wisdom of leaders in the fields of nutrition, fitness, psychology, spirituality and personal development and have outlined the main ideas providing a framework for you to choose what works best for you to develop your own healthy lifestyle. If you struggle with living a sedentary life, weight issues, pain or if you simply don't feel well, then this plan will guide you in becoming your own health coach.

Secrets of a Good Health Coach

As a health and wellness coach, the most common thoughts I hear from clients are:

- ♥ I don't have time to exercise.
- ♥ I'm too stressed out to do anything about my health right now.
- ♥ Why should I eat something that doesn't taste good?
- ♥ Nobody is going to tell me what to eat.
- ♥ I don't care. It won't make a difference whether I exercise today or not.
- ♥ I'm not going to give up eating the foods I love.

Do you think any of these thoughts? Are they really true? Many people live without thinking consciously. They develop habits without being aware of how the choices they make impact their health. Others beat themselves up about their choices and behaviors. People who ask for the help of a health coach, personal trainer or therapist are usually ready to make positive changes. Whether you choose to seek help or use a guide such as this, start by BEING AWARE, and then determine what you want, set realistic goals and a system of support to help you follow through.

Living a healthy lifestyle is not difficult. Suffering *a heart attack or stroke is difficult. Living with diabetes or pain can be difficult.* The first step is to open your mind to new ways of thinking. Change can seem scary, *but it is not about drastic changes.* Living a healthy lifestyle is an enjoyable journey. *Are you ready to begin?* Focus on what you want, not on what you don't want. Take small steps and change one habit at a time. Affirm your health and well-being now.

> Well-being is not the fruit of something you do;
> It is the essence of who you are.
> There is nothing you need to change,
> do, be or have in order to be happy.
> ~Michael Neill, success coach and author

What are the Secrets of Fit and Healthy People?

Healthy and physically fit people know that reaching a healthy weight does not mean dieting, depriving yourself or beating yourself up. You must care about yourself enough to want to make better choices, however, you do not have to starve or cut out any food groups or spend hours at the gym. Fit and healthy people have learned how to *incorporate good eating habits, activity and relaxation into their daily life. They make healthy habits a part of their everyday life.* What are your barriers to becoming healthy?

- ♥   Do you think you have to make big changes? Are you afraid of change?
- ♥   Do you think eating well requires extra time and money?
- ♥   Do you dislike exercise?
- ♥   Do you want results now and don't want to wait for the end results?

Creating your own healthy lifestyle habits means that you incorporate simple changes that will fit your needs so you want to sustain them for life.

> Self- discipline is doing what you need to even when you don't feel like doing it.
> ~ Brian Tracy

The Leading Causes of Death in the U.S. are Preventable!

When I first learned that *more than 80 to 90%* of all deaths in the United States are *preventable* through lifestyle changes, I was both shocked and relieved. It was the first time that I heard that I was not destined to die young from a heart attack like my relatives, and that by changing my lifestyle habits; I can live longer with a better quality of life! This is great news. We can do something to prevent illness and premature aging! Being sedentary and obese leads to many illnesses including heart disease, certain cancers and type 2 diabetes, which is an epidemic in America. Children are rapidly becoming diagnosed with type 2 diabetes because of poor eating habits and lack of exercise. But there is hope: A study published in the New England Journal of Medicine determined that *more than 90% of type 2 diabetes cases can with prevented by lifestyle changes.*

> We are what we repeatedly do. Excellence, then, is not an act but a habit.
> ~ Aristotle

Most illnesses and injuries in our country are caused from overeating foods that do not nourish our bodies, from stress and from leading sedentary lifestyles. *The solution to most of America's health problems is simple; yet we are so busy that we do not slow down enough to see the answers.* To be healthy, you do not have to give up anything; you simply need to learn how to make balanced choices. The wisdom of "everything in moderation" translates to balance. Before you reach for a pill to solve your aches and pains, to help you lose weight or make you feel happier, remember that you have the power to create a healthy body and mind by eating nutritious foods and moving your body. If you consistently incorporate these steps into your life, you build healthy habits. Being healthy and fit can be easy and it can be done by making one choice at a time.

Know the Numbers that Will Save Your Life

Obesity, type 2 diabetes, high cholesterol, and heart disease are the most urgent health problems facing Americans today. Two-thirds of us are overweight or obese. The Centers for Disease Control states that obesity is linked to high cholesterol, heart disease, high blood pressure, gallstones, complications in pregnancy, infertility, bladder control, depression, stroke, diabetes and some forms of cancer. According to AARP, the brain appears to shrink more and age faster in overweight people.

If you are the type of person who takes care of everyone else before taking care of yourself, then you may not take the time to go to your doctor for your annual health screenings. Make it a priority to get an annual examination and understand your results.

Being knowledgeable about health tests will motivate you to take charge of your health and reduce your risk for disease. Knowing where you stand can save your life.

The Leading Causes of Death in the United States are Lifestyle Related, *Which Means that the American lifestyle is Killing Us.*

Let these words sink in: 80 to 90% of the deaths in the U.S. *can be prevented* with healthy lifestyles! If more people understood that we have the power to prevent illness, we would not have a health care crisis in our country today. Heart disease and stroke alone cost American's billions each year in health care costs and lost productivity. That is just the economic side. When you read these facts, think about the people you love and how it will affect you:

- Every 44 seconds someone in the U.S. has a heart attack. Cardiovascular disease is the leading cause of death in the U.S. and kills roughly the same number of people each year as cancer, lower respiratory diseases and accidents combined. *About half of all U.S. adults (47%) have at least one risk factor for heart disease.*
- Each year about 600,000 people die of heart disease
- Each year more than 795,000 in the U.S. have a stroke
- 87 percent of lung cancer is caused by tobacco use.
- We can avoid up to 90 percent of all cancers according to The American Institute for Cancer Research
- Over 18 million people in the U.S have diabetes-*an increase of epidemic proportions*
- An estimated 79 million adults have pre-diabetes and it *can be prevented.*

♥ **Health Coach Wisdom:** Understanding your health numbers will help motivate you to take action.

Here are some common risk factors for heart disease:

- **High cholesterol levels, High blood pressure**
- **Diabetes, Obesity**
- **Smoking**
- **Lack of physical activity**
- **Age**
- **Family history of heart disease**

What Are Your Numbers?

Talk to your doctor about your numbers. Everybody is different. These numbers are updated and changed often and are intended for a general reference.

Blood Pressure: *Make sure you get your blood pressure screened yearly.*
The top number (systolic pressure) is the pressure that is put on the artery walls when the heart beats. The bottom number (diastolic pressure) represents the pressure on the arteries between heartbeats. *High blood pressure can cause nicks in your arteries, leading to inflammation and dangerous blood clots that cause heart attacks and strokes.*

115/75 is ideal
120/80 is normal
140/90 or above is high

Cholesterol: The numbers you need to focus on are: total cholesterol, the HDL ("healthy") LDL ("lousy") cholesterol, which leads to cholesterol buildup in the arteries), and *triglycerides (fats in the bloodstream).*

Total cholesterol should be less than 200.

HDL levels at 60 or above are desirable and can even reduce heart disease; levels below 40 can increase risk.

LDL levels are near ideal at 100-129. Any number above 130 is borderline high to high. People who are at risk for heart disease should aim for below 100.

Triglycerides should be below 150.

Blood Sugar-Fasting Glucose: This is a measure of how much sugar (glucose) is in your blood. High blood sugar can signal diabetes which increases your risk of heart disease according to Tracy Stevens, MD, a New York Cardiologist and spokesperson for the American Heart Association.

What is normal?

- Levels below 100 are normal (80-90 preferred)
- Levels between 100-125 are considered pre-diabetes *and need to be lowered;*
- Levels 126 or higher typically results in a diabetes diagnosis.

A1C *(test measuring your blood sugar over a few months)* should be 5.6% or less.

Are you at risk for diabetes? If you are overweight, have high blood pressure, or a family history, *ask your doctor if you should get a blood sugar test now.* The American Diabetes Association reports 79 million people in the U.S. are pre-diabetic.

Body Mass Index (BMI): Less than 25 is recommended. This number, based on a calculation of height and weight, determines whether or not a person is overweight or obese. *See the chart on following page for your number. (The BMI Chart is not always an accurate indicator if you are physically fit, as muscle weighs more than fat.)*

Normal: BMI of 18.5 to 24.9
Overweight: 25 to 29.9
30 or higher is considered obese.

Waist circumference: The number of inches around your unclothed abdomen, just above your hip bone. *(The narrowest part of your torso)* Larger waistlines have been linked to higher risk of disease because of the fat's proximity to your organs.

For women, a waist measurement of 35 inches (89 centimeters) or more indicates an unhealthy concentration of belly fat and a greater risk of problems such as heart disease, high blood pressure and type 2 diabetes.

For men, a waist measurement of 40 inches (102 centimeters) or more is considered cause for concern. Over 35 inches for women and over 40 inches for men are considered strong indicators of abdominal obesity.

Waist to Hip Ratio: The location of excess body fat is significant. People who gain weight in the abdominal area are at an increased risk of developing coronary heart disease, high blood pressure, diabetes and stroke compared to those who gain weight in the hip area. A quick and reliable technique for determining body-fat distribution is the waist to hip circumference ratio. *To calculate, divide your waist measurement by your hip measurement.*

Classification	Men	Women
High Risk	>1.0	>.85
Moderate Risk	0.90-1.0	0.80-.085
Lower Risk	<0.90	<0.80

♥ **Health Coach Wisdom:** Your first step in creating a healthy lifestyle is to make an appointment with your doctor to get a full check up with blood tests and ask for the results. Keep a file with your medical numbers so you have a baseline to start from and understand your goal numbers to shoot for.

The choices you make are either causing you to *age prematurely* or *helping you* to live longer. You can't stop aging, but you can control reduce your risk for disease and how you feel. Here are the areas where you can take control:

- **Reduce aging and inflammation of your heart and blood vessels** which can cause strokes, heart attacks, memory loss and impotence
- **Reduce aging of your immune system** which can lead to autoimmune diseases, infection and cancer
- **Reduce aging caused by environmental issues** and how you react to life

Your risk factors are determined by such things as your age, family and medical history. *Why should you bother to understand your health numbers? Because ignoring them could be fatal.* The numbers from your medical tests are predictors of your likelihood of developing illness such as Cardiovascular Disease.

Atherosclerosis is a process in which fatty deposits of cholesterol and calcium accumulate on the walls of the arteries, causing them to harden, thicken and lose elasticity. If the vessels that supply blood to the heart are narrowed, the blood supply is limited and the increased oxygen demand by the heart cannot be met. This can result in chest discomfort, called angina, and possibly a heart attack. Angina can feel like a pressure or tightness in the chest, or in the arm, shoulder or jaw. This pain may be accompanied by shortness of breath, sweating, nausea, palpitations or racing heart.

Locate your height and weight on the Body Mass Index Chart to find your health classification:

Body Mass Index Table

	Normal						Overweight					Obese										Extreme Obesity														
BMI	19	20	21	22	23	24	25	26	27	28	29	30	31	32	33	34	35	36	37	38	39	40	41	42	43	44	45	46	47	48	49	50	51	52	53	54
Height (inches)												Body Weight (pounds)																								
58	91	96	100	105	110	115	119	124	129	134	138	143	148	153	158	162	167	172	177	181	186	191	196	201	205	210	215	220	224	229	234	239	244	248	253	258
59	94	99	104	109	114	119	124	128	133	138	143	148	153	158	163	168	173	178	183	188	193	198	203	208	212	217	222	227	232	237	242	247	252	257	262	267
60	97	102	107	112	118	123	128	133	138	143	148	153	158	163	168	174	179	184	189	194	199	204	209	215	220	225	230	235	240	245	250	255	261	266	271	276
61	100	106	111	116	122	127	132	137	143	148	153	158	164	169	174	180	185	190	195	201	206	211	217	222	227	232	238	243	248	254	259	264	269	275	280	285
62	104	109	115	120	126	131	136	142	147	153	158	164	169	175	180	186	191	196	202	207	213	218	224	229	235	240	246	251	256	262	267	273	278	284	289	295
63	107	113	118	124	130	135	141	146	152	158	163	169	175	180	186	191	197	203	208	214	220	225	231	237	242	248	254	259	265	270	278	282	287	293	299	304
64	110	116	122	128	134	140	145	151	157	163	169	174	180	186	192	197	204	209	215	221	227	232	238	244	250	256	262	267	273	279	285	291	296	302	308	314
65	114	120	126	132	138	144	150	156	162	168	174	180	186	192	198	204	210	216	222	228	234	240	246	252	258	264	270	276	282	288	294	300	306	312	318	324
66	118	124	130	136	142	148	155	161	167	173	179	186	192	198	204	210	216	223	229	235	241	247	253	260	266	272	278	284	291	297	303	309	315	322	328	334
67	121	127	134	140	146	153	159	166	172	178	185	191	198	204	211	217	223	230	236	242	249	255	261	268	274	280	287	293	299	306	312	319	325	331	338	344
68	125	131	138	144	151	158	164	171	177	184	190	197	203	210	216	223	230	236	243	249	256	262	269	276	282	289	295	302	308	315	322	328	335	341	348	354
69	128	135	142	149	155	162	169	176	182	189	196	203	209	216	223	230	236	243	250	257	263	270	277	284	291	297	304	311	318	324	331	338	345	351	358	365
70	132	139	146	153	160	167	174	181	188	195	202	209	216	222	229	236	243	250	257	264	271	278	285	292	299	306	313	320	327	334	341	348	355	362	369	376
71	136	143	150	157	165	172	179	186	193	200	208	215	222	229	236	243	250	257	265	272	279	286	293	301	308	315	322	329	338	343	351	358	365	372	379	386
72	140	147	154	162	169	177	184	191	199	206	213	221	228	235	242	250	258	265	272	279	287	294	302	309	316	324	331	338	346	353	361	368	375	383	390	397
73	144	151	159	166	174	182	189	197	204	212	219	227	235	242	250	257	265	272	280	288	295	302	310	318	325	333	340	348	355	363	371	378	386	393	401	408
74	148	155	163	171	179	186	194	202	210	218	225	233	241	249	256	264	272	280	287	295	303	311	319	326	334	342	350	358	365	373	381	389	396	404	412	420
75	152	160	168	176	184	192	200	208	216	224	232	240	248	256	264	272	279	287	295	303	311	319	327	335	343	351	359	367	375	383	391	399	407	415	423	431
76	156	164	172	180	189	197	205	213	221	230	238	246	254	263	271	279	287	295	304	312	320	328	336	344	353	361	369	377	385	394	402	410	418	426	435	443

Source: Adapted from Clinical Guidelines on the Identification, Evaluation, and Treatment of Overweight and Obesity in Adults: The Evidence Report.

♥ **Health Coach Wisdom:** Three 20 minute work outs per week will strengthen your heart and help you live longer. Even walking just 10 minutes a day lowers your LDL (*lousy cholesterol*) raises your HDL, (*healthy cholesterol*) and decreases inflammation. Aim for 30 to 45 minutes five days per week or 150 minutes or more total. *Walking 30 minutes five to seven days a week significantly decreases your risk of dying from heart disease.*

Metabolic syndrome is the name for a group of risk factors linked to overweight and obesity including excessive fat around the abdomen, elevated blood pressure, blood glucose, triglycerides, and lower levels of the good HDL cholesterol. These factors increase your risk of coronary artery disease and other health problems, such as diabetes and stroke. You can develop any one of these risk factors by itself, but they tend to occur together. Metabolic Syndrome can make you feel tired, depressed, irritable and somewhat confused. It is a dangerous condition and may even increase the incidence of cancer.

Research shows that most people with pre-diabetes will develop diabetes—*if not stopped*. Diabetes, like heart disease, is a silent killer. The good news is that pre-diabetes doesn't have to progress to diabetes. There are steps you can take to control your blood sugar now to reduce your risk for developing diabetes and minimize your risk of all health complications.

The Diabetes Prevention Program Proves that Preventing Type 2 Diabetes is Possible

The original Diabetes Prevention Program (DPP) was a research study funded by the National Institutes of Health (NIH) and supported by the Centers for Disease Control and Prevention (CDC). The results showed that making certain lifestyle changes and continuing them over time can prevent type 2 diabetes in people who are at risk. In the original group, participants cut their risk for type 2 diabetes by 58%. People over sixty cut their risk by 71%.

I was fortunate enough to be a part of the National Diabetes Prevention Program where I taught the program for over two years. During that time period, working with many groups of people, only one person passed over to the diabetes blood sugar range. We taught simple lifestyle changes such as increased walking and physical activity, improving eating habits and reducing stress. The biggest take home message is: *even small changes can have big rewards for your health!*

A study by Joslin Diabetes Center researchers showed that obese adults who lost just 7% of their body weight and did moderate exercise, such as walking, for six months improved their major blood vessel function by approximately 80% regardless of whether or not they have type 2 diabetes. If you weigh 200 pounds that means losing just fourteen pounds will yield life saving results!

People make achieving wellness too hard.
~ Becky Captain, Nurse Practitioner

Learn the Unexpected Warning Signs of a Heart Attack

♥ **Health Coach Wisdom:** One in three deaths in the United States is caused by cardiovascular disease. 80 to 90% of heart disease can be prevented through diet and lifestyle.

Heart disease- the number one killer in America- affects women as well as men. According to the American Heart Association (AHA), heart disease kills more than 500,000 women annually and often presents itself differently in women than it does in men. It is imperative that we learn the traditional warning signs of a heart attack which include chest discomfort, shortness of breath and pain in one or both arms. Pay special attention to the less common signs: shortness of breath, nausea or jaw pain. Additionally, as the U.S. population ages and obesity increases, more strokes are occurring. Maintaining a healthy lifestyle can cut your risk for first-time stroke by 80 percent, according to new guidelines from the American Heart Association and the American Stroke Association.

One Sunday afternoon in August 1991, my phone rang. I had taken my three-year-old son and eight-month-old baby boy over to my mother's house earlier that morning so that she could spend the day with her grandchildren. When I answered the phone, my mother told me she wasn't feeling well, and asked me to come over. When I arrived at her house, I found her clammy and out of breath. She said her stomach hurt, and I thought she had the flu. She grabbed her abdomen and told me she was in pain. My mother rarely got sick, so I was worried and told her we needed to call a doctor. My mother didn't have a family doctor because she believed that she took good care of her health.

After a few minutes, her pain became unbearable. I grabbed the phone book and begin looking for a doctor. Being a Sunday, I dialed the number of an emergency doctor. I spoke to the doctor and recited my mother's symptoms: nausea, abdominal pain and clammy skin. He told me to go to the store and get her an antacid. I then proceeded to make the biggest mistake of my life; I left my baby boys with my sick mother and ran to the store. When I returned, I found my mother doubled over in pain and then made another life changing mistake, I put the boys in the car with my mom, took the extra time to go to my house to leave them with my husband and then nearly two hours after my mother originally called me, I drove her to the hospital. For several hours, the doctors did not know what was wrong, but they later told me she was having a heart attack and that they were waiting for the on-call cardiologist to show up and administer a clot busting drug. When he arrived, he told me it was too late to give her the drug, too much time had passed and too much damage and been done to her heart. She survived, but she did not live long and was never the same lovely, energetic woman again. She was only sixty-two years old.

Twenty three years ago, my family was not aware that smoking and eating foods high in saturated fat contributed to heart disease. While my mom thought she ate healthful foods, she also ate foods high in saturated fat. In addition, she struggled with quitting smoking. She gained and lost weight, was active, *yet had no formal exercise program.* She was a woman who took care of and worried about everyone else—*except herself.*

Like my mom, most people do not equate their lifestyle with positive or negative effects on their body. They don't know that it is very bad for your heart to lose and gain weight often. Each time you make a choice, take time to think about how it affects your heart, your arteries, your brain and ultimately your loved ones.

Life Saving Tips from the American Heart Association

If you or someone you know shows signs of heart attack or stroke, call 9-1-1 right away. An Emergency Medical Services (EMS) team can begin treatment upon arrival. That means treatment can begin sooner than it would if the patient arrived at the hospital by car. What's more, the EMS team is also trained to revive someone whose heart has stopped, saving hundreds of lives each year. If you have symptoms and you cannot access EMS, ask someone to drive you to the hospital immediately. Do not drive yourself, unless there's no other option.

One Meal Affects the Health of Your Arteries

"Plaque starts inside the artery wall, is inflamed and if it bursts can produce a heart attack," says Becky K. Captain, RN, MSN, CLS, BC, FNP-C, and a certified Family Nurse Practitioner who specializes in Preventive Cardiology. "When we exercise it creates a protective cap over the plaque helping to reduce the risk of heart attacks. If you have risk factors, please see your doctor and begin a healthy lifestyle program to reduce your risks. People make healthy living difficult when it really is very simple" she told me during an interview. "Plaque contains fat, cholesterol and other substances, which can grow large enough to significantly reduce blood flow through an artery. One meal affects the health of your arteries," according to Becky Captain, "one high-fat meal does narrow your arteries for about six hours. Meals high in saturated fat such as cheeseburgers, ice cream and french fries...*that is the kind of meal heart attacks are made of.*"

What Is Stroke?

Stroke is the fourth-leading cause of death in the United States and a leading cause of disability. It is a type of vascular disease that affects the arteries leading to and within the brain. A stroke occurs when an artery that carries blood, oxygen and nutrients to the brain either bursts or is blocked by a clot. When that happens, part of the brain can't get the blood (and oxygen) it needs, so it starts to die.

> *Upon my mother's release from the hospital after her heart attack, I would stop by and visit her. One morning, I arrived to find her acting peculiar. When I asked her questions, she just looked at me without answering. She couldn't speak, but looked fine. I called her cardiologist, who told me to bring her into his office. When we arrived, he told me to drive her straight to the hospital—she had a stroke. I did not know the warning signs; if I did, I could have called 911 immediately. Fortunately, she survived for a while, but even further damage was done.*

When part of the brain dies from lack of blood flow, the part of the body it controls is affected. Strokes can cause paralysis, affect language and vision, among other problems. Seeking early treatment can minimize the potentially devastating effects of stroke. We must be able to recognize the warning signs and act quickly.

> *My mother lived for five more months before passing away from congestive heart failure due to her heart attack and stroke. At sixty-two she left behind a family of daughters, sons-in-law, grandchildren, friends and relatives who depended on her for her love and support. She missed weddings, births, graduations, and every event of our lives. We have all missed out on her wisdom and guidance, just because we did not know about heart disease or the warning signs. Please learn from this real and very painful story so you can prevent this from happening to you or someone you love.*

Learn the Signs of Stroke

FAST is an acronym to help you remember the signs of stroke:

Face drooping
Arm weakness (numbness or weakness in face, arm or leg)
Speech difficulty (confusion, trouble speaking or understanding)
Time to call 911

The Silent Killer: Diabetes

Insulin is a hormone your cells need to store and use energy from food. Insulin is responsible for getting glucose into your cells. If you have diabetes, insulin is not able to do its job, which causes glucose to build up in your blood. High levels of glucose then circulate through your body, damaging cells along the way.

There are three Types of Diabetes: **Type 1 Diabetes** (also referred to as Juvenile or Insulin-dependent Diabetes): The pancreas cannot make insulin or makes very little. **Type 2 Diabetes** (also called Adult-onset Diabetes): The pancreas produces insulin, but it does not make enough or your body doesn't use the insulin it makes. Type 2 develops slowly. Eight in ten people with this type of diabetes are overweight. Type 2 Diabetes is becoming more common in children and teenagers due to the increase in obesity. **Gestational Diabetes:** The cause is unknown but may be the result of hormones during pregnancy blocking the action of insulin.

Symptoms of diabetes include: Frequent urination, excessive thirst, weight loss, feeling tired, irritability, blurred vision, frequent illness or infection, poor circulation (tingling or numbness in the feet or hands). *If you think you may have diabetes, consult a doctor now.*

♥ **Health Coach Wisdom:** Type 2 diabetes can be prevented. Even if you have been diagnosed with pre-diabetes, you can lower your blood sugar by seeking help and help prevent diabetes by losing only 7% of your body weight and participating in activities such as walking for thirty minutes five times per week.

Why Should You Quit Smoking?

The morning my mother died, five months after her heart attack, the doctor came out to the hospital waiting room and told us she was gone. Her heart had been damaged too severely. He also told us "If your mother hadn't smoked, she would be alive right now." I knew at that moment I had to do something to warn other people. I could not help her, but if you are a smoker, maybe this book can help you take action to quit smoking.

Smokers have a higher risk of developing many chronic disorders, including cancer and atherosclerosis, the buildup of fatty substances in the arteries which can lead to coronary heart disease, heart attack and stroke. Smoking is the most preventable cause of premature death in the United States.

Prevention is the Key to a Healthy Heart

There are many ways you can prevent heart disease *even if you have a family history.*

The American Heart Association recommends having a few meatless meals each week and increasing the amount of fiber and whole grains in your diet by eating more plant foods. There are many ways to accomplish this. See Chapter nine and ten for ways to eat more plant foods, such as oatmeal, barley, quinoa, brown rice, beans, lentils, nuts, seeds, soy, vegetables and fruit. Plant foods contain fiber with no cholesterol. Animal foods do not have fiber, while they do contain cholesterol. Manage your weight, blood pressure and cholesterol. *Here are some proven strategies to help you take control of your heart health:*

- ♥ Exercise on a consistent basis
- ♥ Read food labels to understand what you are eating
- ♥ Get sufficient sleep
- ♥ Ask your doctor about nutritional supplements
- ♥ Watch your weight, blood pressure and cholesterol
- ♥ Sleep well
- ♥ Stop smoking

It takes a Healthy Body to have a Healthy Mind and Vice Versa

People who are pessimistic, who worry and live in fear have hormonal responses that lead to heart disease. Learning to relax and be calm is something you *can learn to do.* If you find yourself feeling angry or stressed out, immediately change your environment. Do something relaxing. Take a walk and practice deep breathing. Yoga, Chi Kung and meditation are proven methods of calming your nervous system and aiding in the prevention of heart disease. If you need help, consider going to a therapist or getting a certified wellness coach for support.

The Choices You Make Affect Other People

When you take care of yourself you inspire others to do so. Conversely, when you overeat, drink too much, and find reason not to exercise, you influence others in that direction. Setting a good example for others is a powerful tool for finding purpose and helping you heal your heart.

♥ **Health Coach Reminder:** Make an appointment with your doctor for your annual physical exam. Write down your results.

My Health Numbers:

Height: _____   Weight: _____
Body Mass Index: _____   Waist Circumference: _____
Blood Pressure: _____   Blood Sugar (Fasting blood glucose: _____
Total Cholesterol: _____   HDL: _____ LDL: _____

Action Steps: This week I will take the following action to protect my health: *(Examples: I will make an appointment with my doctor, I will quit smoking, or I will write down my vision and an affirmation for this month.)*

My Action Plan Goal for Chapter One is:

_____Target Date: _____

The steps I will take to achieve my health goal are:

• _____
• _____
• _____

On my website you will find an Action Plan form and ideas that you can download for twelve months of healthy habits to create your healthy lifestyle. Visit www.lynellross.com for more information about wellness coaching.

Recommended Resources:

- American Heart Association www.heart.org. **To take a heart assessment**, go to www.mylifecheck.heart.org.
- American Diabetes Association www.diabetes.org
- American Cancer Society www.cancer.org
- American Red Cross www.redcross.org
- Mayo Clinic www.mayoclinic.com

Books for further inspiration:

Supercoach, 10 Secrets to Transform Anyone's Life, by Michael Neill, Hay House Inc. 2009

I Can Do It~How to Use Affirmations to Change Your Life by Louise L. Hay, Hay House Inc. 2004, Includes an affirmation CD.

10 Secrets for Success and Inner Peace by Dr. Wayne Dyer, Hay House, Inc. 2001

The Dragon Doesn't Live Here Anymore-Living Fully, Loving Freely by Alan Cohen, Random House, 1990

You Can Create an Exceptional Life by Louise Hay & Cheryl Richardson, Richardson Enterprises, Inc. and Louise L. Hay, Hay House, Inc. 2011.

Chapter 2

It's Easy to Eat Well:
The Healing Power of Good Nutrition

♥ **Health Coach Secret:** Focus your attention on the benefits of good nutrition to prevent disease, improve your brain power, brighten your mood and help you thrive.

What you eat has everything to do with the way you feel and how healthy you are.

One of the reasons I decided to write this book was to share the discovery I made while researching what to eat. Feeling powerless over the heart disease that had attacked everyone in my family, I was astonished to find that we have the ability to prevent heart disease and illnesses such as type 2 diabetes and many forms of cancer by improving our lifestyles and eating habits. I learned how to prepare foods that are satisfying and taste great! I found a simple way to eat foods I love, *maintain my healthy body weight* and feel great. You can do it too.

You Can Develop Nutritional Fitness

By giving your body the nutrition it needs in the correct portions, you can enjoy what you eat while appreciating food for the gift that it is. Real, fresh whole food is a treasure. We have learned to feel guilty about eating instead of respecting quality food. Everywhere we turn there is something available to eat, yet most of what's readily available and being *marketed to us* isn't real food, and it certainly isn't nutritious. Most restaurant chains serve pre-prepared and processed foods.

If it comes from a package, is manufactured with dyes or preservatives, or is mixed with ingredients you cannot pronounce, then you may want to consider what you are putting in your body. Many Americans are either overweight, have diabetes, or other diseases, while at the same time suffering from malnutrition. Even at the correct weight one can still be *malnourished*. This is a health crisis that can be remedied. Starting with a positive attitude toward learning *what to eat* and *how much to eat*, we can enjoy delicious foods and be stronger than ever.

Eating Well Leads to a High Quality Life

The health you enjoy is largely your choice.
~ Abraham Lincoln

Caring about your health and the long term quality of your life enables you to make better choices. If you eat well and choose nutritious foods, but weigh more than you would like, *you are simply eating too much and probably not getting enough physical activity.*

The choices you make today are going to impact the way you sleep tonight, the way you feel tomorrow and the results at your next medical check-up. Good choices today may prevent a stroke, a heart attack, diabetes or cancer tomorrow. If you see the way you eat and prepare your food as a pleasurable experience rather than an ordeal, your attitude about food may shift. Eating foods that are fresh, and good for you is easy and rewarding. Educating yourself about what to eat is crucial because you must make choices for yourself. Statistics prove that people who eat the recommended portions from the food groups tend to live longer and healthier lives.

Change the Way You Think About Your Health
To Achieve the Well-Being You Desire

♥ **Health Coach Wisdom:** If you want to feel good, and reach a healthy weight, YOU MUST EAT. People skip meals and starve themselves because they think they are overweight and don't deserve to eat, or they are too busy. You set yourself up for failure by skipping meals. Eat breakfast, lunch, healthy snacks, and dinner to maintain a healthy weight, keep your energy high and your mood happy.

The beauty in living a healthy lifestyle is that you get to create the life you want, one choice at a time. Think before you eat, purchase food or dine out. Making a meal plan will help you to eat more nutritional foods. Dr. Linda Page in her book, *"Diets for Healthy Healing"* explains the benefits of eating well:

> Wholesome food not only fuels your body, but it can help you solve your health problems. Your diet can keep your energy levels up and stress levels down; your skin, hair and nails healthy; your complexion glowing; your eyes bright; and your bones and muscles strong. It can fine tune mental awareness and prevent disease from taking hold. A poor diet and junk foods produce lethargy, illness and indifference. Good food is good medicine. It is the prime factor for changing your body chemically and psychologically. The food you eat changes your weight, your mood, the texture and look of your body, your outlook on life, indeed the entire universe for you...and therefore your future.

In this chapter you will find a simple eating plan based on nutrition customized to your own tastes and needs. It is not difficult to follow and will easily become a part of your daily life. In other words, *you will be creating your own healthy lifestyle.* To achieve your health goals, decide to take action. Set your priorities now and follow through to become healthy and fit.

Get Back To Basics

Whether you have a weight problem or not, food affects the way you feel and determines the state of your health. If you have weight issues, they may stem from the way you *think* about food and weight loss. Before making a shift toward healthy eating, you must first decide why it is important for you to attain a healthy weight or optimize your health. Is it that you want feel better and have a good quality of life? Have you been confused by advertisements? Many advertisers tell us that eating well is hard, that weight loss is difficult without the aid of pills or exercise gadgets. This is simply not true. You can develop a healthy, effective eating plan and a lifestyle that that will provide the nutrition you need from foods you enjoy!

I have researched nutrition information from The American Heart Association, The Academy of Nutrition and Dietetics, The United States Department of Agriculture, The Center for Science in the Public Interest, Dr. Andrew Weil, and Dr. Dean Ornish's work on reversing heart disease. I have discovered that whole fresh foods, fruits, vegetables, whole grains, lean proteins, and fat-free or low-fat dairy provide the nutrition most of us need. However, you need to learn what is best for your body, and your health. To begin, shop for wholesome foods and eat them in the proper portions. Here is a simple plan to get you started:

Power to Be Healthy Eating Action Plan

Think nutrition and eat from food groups: Choose nutritious foods and follow the suggested food groups from The USDA My Plate or the Mediterranean Food Guide. Strive to get the recommended amounts of fruits, vegetables, whole grains, dairy, leans meats/ poultry/fish /beans, nuts/legumes and oils, *the fresher the better. Reduce consumption of red meats and full- fat dairy, unhealthy fats and refined carbohydrates such as products made with white flour and white sugar.*

Eat proper portion sizes. Read the charts in this chapter to learn your recommended amounts and portion sizes in terms of cups, half cups, tablespoons and teaspoons. *Portion size is the most important key to weight loss or maintaining your weight!*

Stabilize your blood sugar to avoid hunger: When you eat nutritious foods in the correct amounts, your blood sugar stabilizes, you won't be hungry and you will feel better.

Eat 3 small meals and 2 or 3 snacks on a routine: Refer to the "my plate" picture in this chapter when you eat a meal. If you eat at approximately the same meal and snack times daily, you will create a routine and will not be hungry because you will give your body the nutrition it needs.

Drink water throughout the day: Adequate hydration is crucial to your health and digestion.

Plan ahead so you know what you will eat for daily meals and snacks. If you eat out, ask for nutritional information so you can be informed.

Grocery shop so you have healthy foods on hand, allowing you to quickly prepare meals and snacks. Read food labels and choose items with few ingredients.

Be grateful for your food. Slow down and enjoy each meal or snack consciously. Be mindful of every bite you eat.

> If you follow these steps, you will create and maintain a
> healthy body, a healthy weight, a healthy mind.

♥ **Health Coach Wisdom:** If you think you are hungry, ask yourself if you are really hungry or if your appetite was triggered by something you saw or smelled. A desire for food does not always mean you are hungry. Drink a glass of water and the urge to eat will usually pass.

How to Achieve Optimal Health Through Better Nutrition

If you have poor eating habits, you are more likely to be unfit, have low energy and develop lifestyle related diseases such as heart disease, diabetes, cancer and obesity. Did you know that anxiety and depression can be caused from a lack of proper nutrients? Take control now by making wise food choices. The *Dietary Guidelines for Americans* emphasizes three major goals for Americans:

- Balance calories with physical activity to manage weight
- Eat more fruits and vegetables, whole grains, fat-free or low-fat dairy products and seafood
- Consume fewer foods with sodium (salt), saturated fats, trans-fats, cholesterol, added sugars and refined grains.

Most people want to eat well, but they don't know how. The first step is to learn about nutrition so you can make your plan. I developed the healthy recipes in this book by learning to substitute unhealthy fats with healthier ones, by reducing sodium and sugar and replacing them with more flavor, spices, and herbs. *Each recipe lists the number of servings, the serving size and food group.* Now let's focus on what to eat *and why.*

What is Nutrition?

Nutrients are life-sustaining substances in food. They work together to supply our bodies with energy and materials to regulate growth, maintenance and repair of body tissues. Vital to our health and survival, the six major classes of nutrients are:

1. Proteins
2. Carbohydrates
3. Fats
4. Vitamins
5. Minerals
6. Water

Protein, carbohydrate and fat are the three nutrients that provide calories. These calories are used by the body to maintain body temperature, and to facilitate the growth and repair of all organs and tissue. Many people are confused and think of carbohydrates and fats as bad. In reality, both serve a vital purpose in our diet. Eating too much of *anything* causes excess weight gain. Fat is a very concentrated source of energy and contains twice the calories of protein and carbohydrate. (*See the breakdown of caloric values below.*) Combine that fact with the problem that deep fried foods soak up great amounts of fat and you have a very high calorie food. It is a triple threat if it is fried in hydrogenated oil or lard.

Carbohydrates, fat and protein are all fuel for the body. Energy is measured in calories. The energy released from the carbohydrates, fat and protein can all be measured in calories. The amount of energy a food provides depends on each of these.

When broken down they provide the following:

Breakdown of Caloric Values

➢ 1 gram protein = 4 calories
➢ 1 gram carbohydrate= 4 calories
➢ 1 gram fat = 9 calories
➢ 1 gram alcohol = 7 calories

What does this mean for you? First, alcohol is not considered to be a nutrient because it does not contribute to the growth, maintenance or repair of body tissue and it is easily converted into fat when caloric intake exceeds output. The process by which nutrients are broken down to yield energy is known as *metabolism.* Your body uses nutrients to fuel all its activities. *The highest source of calories comes from fat and alcohol.* In the chapter we will learn about *healthy fats* that our bodies need and how to reduce the unhealthy types of fat that can lead to heart disease and type 2 diabetes. We will also learn to differentiate between unhealthy carbohydrates and healthier carbohydrates that give us the energy we need to move.

Essential Nutrients

If you are not feeling well, chances are you are not getting the nutrition you need. You can nourish yourself back to good health! The body has the ability to make certain nutrients from other nutrients; however, *there are some compounds that the body cannot make for itself.* We call these essential because they are absolutely indispensable for bodily functions and we need to get them from food sources outside our body. There are about 40 essential nutrients to be concerned about. It is simple to get all the essential nutrients in appropriate amounts by eating a variety from the food groups.

Recommended Nutrient Intakes – What to Eat

How do you know what to eat? Normal healthy adults of average size and who engage in physical activity should consume the following amounts of nutrients daily to remain in optimal health:

Protein: Approximately 50-70 grams, depending on body size, or 12 to 20% of caloric intake. **Protein foods are: beef, pork, chicken, fish, nuts, eggs, dairy products, tofu, whole grains & legumes (plants of the bean and pea family)** *Make lean choices and prepare with little or no added fat. Cut back or eliminate fatty cuts of beef and pork.*

- Protein builds and repairs body tissues, muscles, ligaments and tendons. Protein is also a major component of enzymes, hormones and antibodies and is important for transporting fluid and energy.
- Proteins are made up of specific combinations of 20 amino acids. *Eight of these amino acids cannot be made in the body and must be supplied by the diet.*

Carbohydrates: A minimum of 125 grams, optimal 350 to 400 grams or 55 to 65% of caloric intake as carbohydrate. **Examples include: fruit, vegetables, grains.** *Eat whole grains, reduce or eliminate white flour and refined carbohydrates.*

- Carbohydrates are essential for muscular performance, brain and central nervous system.
- Carbohydrates provide a major source of fuel to the body
- Carbohydrates provide dietary fiber to keep digestion moving

Fats: Approximately 30 to 65 grams, depending on caloric consumption or 25 to 30% of caloric intake from fat. **Healthy examples are olive oil, flax, trans-fat free buttery spreads and unsaturated oils that occur naturally in foods such as avocados, fatty fish, nuts, olives, seeds and shellfish.** *Fats to limit or avoid: mayonnaise, salad dressings, margarine and fatty cuts of meat.* Fat does provide essential fatty acids which are necessary for the proper functioning of cell membranes, skin, and hormones and for transporting fat-soluble vitamins.

- Fats are the chief storage form of energy in the body
- Fats insulate and protect vital organs

Saturated Fat – 7-10% or less of caloric intake from fat, *such as cheese, butter, visible fat.*

Vitamins – *Specific amounts are listed in the Recommended Dietary Allowances (RDA)* visit www.nutrition.gov.

- Vitamins help promote and regulate chemical reactions and bodily processes
- Vitamins help to release energy from food

Minerals – Specific amounts are listed in the RDA

- Minerals enable enzymes to function
- Minerals are a component of hormones
- Minerals are a part of bone and nerve impulses

Water – 2-3 quarts per day

- About 60% of the body is composed of water
- Water is essential for life as we cannot store or conserve it

  1 cup = 8 ounces
  2 cups = 16 ounces or a pint
  4 cups = 32 ounces or 1 quart
  8 cups = 64 ounces or 2 quarts
  12 cups = 96 ounces or 3 quarts

Why Drink Water?

Water is essential to good health. Needs vary by individual so your water needs depend on many factors, including your health, your activity level and where you live. Every day you lose water through your breath, perspiration, urine and bowel movements. For your body to function properly, you must replenish its water supply by consuming beverages and foods that contain water. Did you know that most of us are chronically dehydrated?

- ♥ Even mild dehydration will slow down your metabolism
- ♥ Lack of water is the number one cause of fatigue
- ♥ Adequate water will ease joint pain and promotes healthy digestion
- ♥ Drinking water can boost memory and clear up fuzzy thinking
- ♥ Dehydration is a leading cause of migraine headaches

How Much Water Do You Need?

A healthy adult living in a temperate climate needs about 8 or 9 cups. Remember:

- **Eight 8-ounce glasses of water or more each day.**
- **Exercise:** If you exercise or sweat, you need to drink extra water.
- **Environment:** In hot or humid weather, you need to drink additional water to help lower your body temperature and replace water lost through sweating.

Water transports nutrients, carries away waste assisting good digestion, moistens eyes, mouth, nose and skin, ensures adequate blood volume and helps maintain normal body temperature.

Dietary Guidelines

This graphic from the USDA shows how we should fill our plate with fruits, grains, vegetables and proteins. For more information visit www.chooseMyPlate.gov.

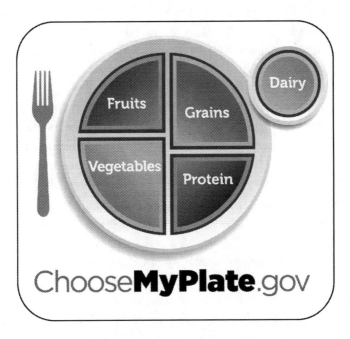

The USDA guidelines provide science-based recommendations to promote health and **reduce risk for major chronic diseases such as cardiovascular disease, type 2 diabetes, hypertension, osteoporosis, certain cancers,** through proper diet and activity. The guidelines are:

1. **Consume adequate nutrients within calorie needs:** *Eat a balanced diet with as many nutrients as possible within the calorie boundaries your body needs.* Limit saturated and trans-fats, cholesterol, added sugars, salt and alcohol.

2. **Promote weight management:** Adults should try to maintain a healthy body weight by balancing calories consumed with calories expended. Those who need to lose weight need to do so in a slow and steady manner.

3. **Incorporate physical activity:**

- All adults should avoid inactivity. Some physical activity is better than none. For substantial health benefits, adults should do at least 150 minutes a week of moderate intensity or 75 minutes of vigorous intensity aerobic activity. Aerobic activity should be performed in bouts of at least 10 minutes throughout the day. To lower your risk for disease, engage in 30 minutes of moderate intensity physical activity most days of the week.

4. **Eat from the food groups** in appropriate amounts: fruits, vegetables, whole grains, fat-free or low-fat dairy products and meats *within caloric requirements.*

5. **Select appropriate fats:** Total fat intake range is between 20-35% of daily calories, with most fats coming from polyunsaturated and monounsaturated sources such as fish, nuts, and vegetable oil. No more than 7-10% of calories from saturated fats.

6. **Select the appropriate carbohydrates:** Fiber rich fruits, vegetables and whole grains. Limit sugars and starch containing foods, such as potatoes and corn. Switch to brown rice and other grains such as quinoa and barley. Choose 100% whole wheat or whole grain bread instead of white.

7. **Balance sodium and potassium consumption.** Americans are advised to choose and prepare foods with little salt and **limit consumption to 2,300 mg** of sodium (about 1 teaspoon of salt) per day. People with high blood pressure, African Americans, and those over 40 should have **no more than 1500 mg per day. Potassium-rich** foods should be consumed to reach 4,700 mg for adults.

8. **Limit alcoholic beverage intake.** Sensible and moderate consumption of alcoholic beverages—defined as no more than on drink per day for women and two drinks per day for men.

9. **Enhance food safety:** Reduce food borne illness by practicing safe recommendations for handling food: Hands, food surfaces, and fruits and vegetables should be washed prior to food prep. Raw, cooked and ready to eat foods should be separated from each other while shopping, preparing and storing them. Foods should be cooked to safe temperatures and perishable food should be refrigerated and/ or defrosted properly. Unpasteurized milk products, juices, raw eggs, sprouts, undercooked or raw meats and poultry should be avoided.

The Food Guide Makes Healthy Eating Easy

The easiest way to eat nutritious foods is to eat from the food groups. Because everyone is different, you must be aware of which foods may affect you or certain medical conditions. Some people have allergies to certain foods or prefer a vegetarian or vegan lifestyle. Learn what is right for you. For the average person, using the food guide plan is an easy and effective method to stay healthy and maintain a naturally healthy weight. You need to understand your own body and choose accordingly.

There are other pyramids that offer health benefits as well. Research shows that the Mediterranean Pyramid offers a healthy approach. Dr. Andrew Weil created an Anti-Inflammatory Food Pyramid and Dr. Dean Ornish created a plan to help combat heart disease. **These plans are based on eating fresh whole foods in proper portions.** For more information to view them on-line go to:

www.choosemyplate.gov : My plate nutritional guidelines
www.oldwayspt.org: The Mediterranean Pyramid
www.drweil.com: Dr. Weil's Anti-Inflammatory Pyramid

The key message is to eat less and move more, to avoid oversized portions and drink water instead of sugary beverages, to eat FEWER foods made from white flour, white sugar and saturated fat. While it is wise to understand the calories in foods, an easy approach is to follow a healthy eating plan by following the number of servings in each of the food groups and eat those servings in the proper portion sizes. If you follow the recommended servings, you will never have to struggle with a weight problem. Most adults fall in the 2,000 calorie range to maintain their weight. The specifics depend on how much you currently weigh and how active you are. In the section on weight loss you will find a simple formula and chart you can use to determine the amount of calories you need each day to maintain your weight. Below is a 2,000 calorie per day plan that you can use and adjust to for your needs:

Sample Daily Plan from the USDA Food Guide at the 2,000 Calorie Level

FOOD GROUP	AMOUNT	SERVING SIZE	EQUIVALENTS
Fruits	2 cups fruit = 4 servings daily	½ cup = 1 medium fruit	½ cup fresh, frozen or canned ¼ cup dried fruit

FOOD GROUP	AMOUNT	SERVING SIZE	EQUIVALENTS
Vegetables Dark Green, Orange Starchy & Legumes	2.5 cups veggies= 5 servings daily	½ cup = ½ cup raw or cooked vegetables	1 cup raw leafy green ½ cup veg. juice
Grains	6 ounces grains **Make at least 3 oz. whole grain**	1 ounce = 1 slice bread 1 cup dry cereal	½ cup cooked rice, pasta, hot cereals
Meat and Beans Nuts, seeds Group	5 ½ ounces daily	1 ounce = 1 egg 1 Tbsp peanut butter or	1 oz. lean meats, poultry, fish ½ ounce nuts, seeds ½ cup cooked beans
Milk Group	3 cups daily	1 cup = 1 cup **low- fat or non-fat** milk/yogurt	1 ½ ounces low- fat or fat-free cheese
Oils	6 teaspoons daily	1 teaspoon = 1 Tsp buttery spread	1 Tbsp light mayonnaise
Discretionary Calorie Allowance "Extras"	267 Calories Solid Fat = 18 grams Added sugar = 8 tsp		1 Tbsp Jam = 3 teaspoons sugar

♥ **Health Coach Wisdom:** To be accurate about what you eat, buy a set of measuring cups and spoons to measure foods you eat at home. You will be surprised how distorted your idea of portions are. Pour yourself a bowl of cereal in the amount you normally eat. Then measure a serving size from the box label. You may be eating from 2 to 4 servings! If you want 2 servings, that is fine, just include it into your daily total. You will have used 2 ounces of your 6 daily ounces. Pour on fat-free or low-fat milk; add a serving of fruit for a balanced meal. *Pick a cereal with 3 grams or more of fiber.*

What to do About Sugar

Almost everyone enjoys the taste of sweets. While there are natural sugars in fruits, milk, vegetables and grains (from foods that provide us with nutrition) it is the use of *added sugars* that we must be careful of. *Added Sugars* are hidden under such names as sucrose, invert sugar, corn sugar, corn syrups, high-fructose corn syrup and honey, to name a few. A food is likely to be high in added sugar if its ingredient list starts with any of these or if they are near the top of the list of ingredients. Added sugar contributes to obesity, type 2 diabetes, arthritis, heart disease and some cancers. Too much sugar causes inflammation in the body! We can enjoy *small amounts* of sugar without harmful effects, but in excess they can be detrimental. The average American eats about 31 teaspoons (124 grams) of sugar every day! Compare this to amounts of added sugars that the USDA Food Guide allows as discretionary calories per day as a *luxury or treat*— and see if you are able to stay at or below these amounts:

- 3 teaspoons for 1600 calorie meal plan
- 5 teaspoons for 1800 calorie meal plan
- 8 teaspoons for 2000 calorie meal plan

Added sugar is a major source of weight gain, obesity, inflammation and other diseases.

♥ **Health Coach Wisdom:** A typical adult can obtain all needed nutrients within about 1500 calories. *Some very active people (athletes and active teenagers) may need up to 3,000 calories per day.* When we eat a slice of 500 calorie chocolate cake or a sweet coffee drink, we use up one forth or more of our daily calories and double the amount of sugar allowed on empty calories.

Sugar is hidden in our food and beverages so it is important for you to READ LABELS. Specifically note the sugar grams in one serving. *To find the number of teaspoons in a serving, divide the grams listed by 4.*

Do the math. Consider what happens when we consume drinks and foods with the following amounts of sugar:

- 12 ounce soda, 38 grams = 10 teaspoons of sugar
- 20 oz. medium soda, 65 grams = 16 teaspoons of sugar
- 36 oz liter of soda, 186 grams = 46 teaspoons of sugar

- 8 oz. Red Bull has 27 grams = 7 teaspoons of sugar
- 16 oz. can lemonade has 48 grams = 7 teaspoons of sugar
- 11 oz. hard lemonade has 30 grams = 7.5 teaspoons of sugar
- Glazed donut has 24 grams of sugar = 6 teaspoons of sugar
- Chocolate candy bar has 28 grams of sugar = 7 teaspoons of sugar
- A slice of chocolate cake has 40 grams of sugar = 10 teaspoons of sugar

Be aware of the amount of sugar when reaching for a beverage or dessert. Read food labels!

♥ **Health Coach Wisdom:** For dessert, make your own the healthy way, not high in saturated fat and sugar, and have a small serving *at least* two hours before bed. Or eat something satisfying with protein such as low-fat yogurt or peanut butter on whole grain crackers or an apple.

Food Groups

Fats & Oils Group

Oils listed in the Food Guide are there because we need them. They are a major source of vitamin E and polyunsaturated fatty acids, including essential fatty acids. Most people get more than enough fat in their diet. We need the healthy types of fats for many reasons. *In contrast*, the solid fats (saturated fat and trans-fats) are listed separately because they are the unhealthy fats are must be limited for *heart health*. Fats are hidden in salad dressings, mayonnaise, foods cooked or fried with butter and oils, and in meat and chicken that have not had the fat and skin trimmed.

To monitor your fat intake, remember to read food labels and look for:

- 1 teaspoon fat = 5 grams
- 3 teaspoons fat = 1 tablespoon or 15 grams
- 4 tablespoons fat = ¼ cup or 60 grams of fat. *It adds up quickly!*

How Saturated Fat is Different than Other Fats

For years we have been warned that saturated fats will clog our arteries. Saturated fats are in butter, whole milk and meats and they harden at room temperature. Newer research has been in the media indicating that saturated fats may not be as harmful as predicted, but it is complicated. A recent study in *the Annals of Internal Medicine* concluded that saturated fat does not appear to increase heart disease risk. *But the news headlines went overboard*. The nutritionists didn't say saturated fat is healthy, the study more reported a lack of harm. Bottom line, the issue is still being studied. Not everyone agrees on how saturated fat impacts our health; some types of saturated fat may be more neutral than others. They are still researching how coconut oil (saturated fat content of 92 percent) and whole milk affects heart disease. It is complicated because foods like beef, dairy, nuts, tropical oils and vegetable oils contain multiple types of saturated and unsaturated fats. It is clear, replacing fat with refined carbohydrates and processed food causes weight gain and a lack of nutrition. Eating too much of any kind of fat also causes weight gain. Be aware of how much and what type of fats you eat, and be the possible affects to your arteries.

So What Do We Eat?

Experts agree that a healthy eating pattern includes fruits, nuts, and vegetables, proper portions of healthy lean proteins like fish, poultry and low-fat or fat-free dairy, minimally processed, whole grain carbohydrates. The guidelines recommend limiting saturated fat to less than 7-10% of total daily calories. Think about the overall quality of your food; make it fresh and whole as much as possible. Key message: *Don't fool yourself into eating a low-fat diet if you are going to fill up on sugar, processed foods and refined carbohydrates.* The bottom line is if you are going to include butter and full fat dairy such as cheese in your meals, do so sparingly. *Everyone agrees* that partially hydrogenated oils do raise your risk of heart disease and should be avoided completely. Read food labels and avoid it.

*We do not need saturated fat. The Dietary Reference Intake from the National Academy of Sciences (DRI) recommendation for 22 grams of sat fat is the **maximum** you should have.*

❤ **Health Coach Wisdom:** *Notice how much extra fat that deep frying adds*: A baked potato has 0 grams of fat. A three-ounce serving of French fries has 15 grams; three ounces of potato chips has 30 grams of fat.

Foods high in saturated fat are also high in calories. These include bacon, fried foods, cheese, fatty meats, marbled steaks, poultry with skin, sausages, pepperoni, ribs, whole milk, cream, whole milk products, cream cheese, ice cream, creamy salad dressings, and butter cream frostings.

The USDA Food Guidelines say we should eat only 5 to 7 teaspoons of fats & oils per day (3 to 4 teaspoons for children ages 2 to 8 years old).

♥ **Health Coach Wisdom:** *We need to limit healthy fats to maintain our weight*: One tablespoon of olive oil has 14 grams of fat that quickly becomes 96 grams of fat if you ladle on ½ cup of salad dressing onto your salad. The calories from fat add up fast. Limit your fats and oils, but don't eliminate them. Healthy Fats sources: nuts, avocados, olive oils, seeds, flax oil and fatty fish.

Grains Group

The USDA food guide measures grains in one-ounce equivalent servings. At least half of your allotment needs to be from whole grains. Aim to eat at least three one-ounce equivalents of whole grains per day. For example *a one-ounce equivalent* includes:

- ½ cup cooked oatmeal, whole-grain pasta, brown rice or barley
- 1 regular slice of 100% whole-grain bread (*look for 100% whole grain*)
- 1 cup of whole-grain ready-to-eat cereal

Here is the take-away message. You get to choose from a variety of options each day, adding up your servings as you go. In one day you could have a serving of oatmeal for breakfast, a sandwich with two slices of bread for lunch and a cup of pasta or rice for dinner and still stay within your 6 ounce allotment. *Choose whole grains for health:* barley, brown rice, bulgur, millet, oats, quinoa, wheat, pasta and popcorn.

Vegetables Group

The daily recommendations for vegetables are to eat more green vegetables like broccoli, kale, chard and spinach. *French fries do not count as a vegetable!* Twelve baby carrots, a large tomato, and two stalks of celery are each equivalent to 1 cup of veggies. Lettuces are measured differently: 2 cups of leafy greens are a serving and are one of the most important foods you can eat for your health. Vegetables help prevent heart disease, certain cancers, type 2 diabetes and provide a variety of vitamins, minerals and anti-oxidants which protect your immune system and aid in digestion.

♥ **Health Coach Wisdom:** Look for new ways to roast, broil, barbeque and sauté vegetables for more flavor. Experiment with spices and herbs to add variety. Eating more vegetables is the key to great health.

Fruits Group

- The recommendation for fruit is in cups. One cup equivalents of fruit are a large banana, peach, orange, 32 grapes, 8 strawberries, or a small apple.

Milk or Dairy Group: Children under the age of 8 need 2 cups of milk per day; for everyone else, 3 cups is the recommendation. It is important for children to drink milk to assist with bone growth. Active youngsters need close to 4 cups of dairy products daily. "There are a lot of people who don't drink milk at all," according to Lona Sandon, RD. They are lacking calcium and vitamin D," she adds, warning that "osteoporosis is a disease you don't see until later in life" but it's linked to lack of calcium and vitamin D early in life. Dairy options equal to 1 cup of milk are 1.5 ounces of hard cheese or 1 cup of yogurt. To prevent heart disease and weight gain, teens and adults should have fat-free or low-fat dairy. *Dairy provides protein.*

Meat/Beans Group

Most people need just 5 to 6.5 ounce equivalents of protein per day: Two ounces of sliced chicken in a salad or sandwich for lunch and a 4-ounce fish filet at dinner. Children under 8 years of age need even less, between 2 and 4 ounces a day.

Keep in mind that the protein in dairy helps contribute to your protein needs. Not everyone eats meat. Vegans and vegetarians use *"meat equivalents."* Beans fill two roles, *as protein sources and as vegetables.* They are measured as ounce equivalents.

- One-quarter cup of cooked beans or peas is a 1-ounce equivalent. That means if you eat a main dish of a cup of lentils or black beans, for instance, you've had 4-ounce equivalents, or almost a full day's requirement. Soy: 2 ounces or a quarter-cup of tofu is a one-ounce equivalent; this includes Tempeh, soybeans, and hummus.

Fish is also in the meat and beans group. While you should avoid fish with high mercury levels such as swordfish, make heart-healthy fish staples of your diet.

- Every ounce of fish counts one for one toward your daily ounce-equivalent protein needs. A 3-ounce can of tuna is a 3-ounce equivalents; a 6-ounce salmon steak is a 6-ounce equivalent.

Nuts and seeds belong to the meat and beans group:

- One-ounce equivalents include 1 tablespoon of peanut butter, 2 tablespoons of hummus, and a half-ounce of nuts or seeds. Remember that nuts are high in calories—*a half-ounce is just seven walnut halves or a dozen almonds*. Because they contain fat, nuts also can count toward the fats and oil category. They are a great source of vitamin E, and are a heart-healthy type of fat. Oils from nuts and other plant sources do not contain cholesterol.

Understanding Food

There are two things that will help you better understand food. The first is in which group a food falls. The second is whether the food contains carbohydrates, protein and/or fat. Some foods contain carbohydrates *and* protein, such as milk, grains, vegetables and fruit. However, meats only contain protein and no carbohydrates.

Carbohydrates: Whole grains, fruits and vegetables are carbohydrates. They include things that are good for us: fiber, vitamins and minerals. "Refined" carbohydrates are processed white bread, white rice, packaged rolls, cookies, crackers etc. *Refined* carbohydrates offer little nutrition or fiber as *all the good vitamins and minerals have been stripped away!*

Proteins: Meat, beans, nuts, seeds, grains, cheese, vegetables, yogurt, milk, cottage cheese, peanut and other nut butters, tofu, soybeans, eggs, poultry and fish. *Vegetables and grains contain protein, but not as much as meat, beans, nuts and milk.* Unprocessed soy is an excellent source of protein. Edamame is a good choice.

Fats & Oils: Fats and oils are necessary, and best from fish, nuts, and vegetable oils. Beware of fats from butter, salad dressings, cheeses, fatty meats, and mayonnaise.

Extras: Limit your intake of "extra" foods. They provide little or no nutrition and lots of fats and sugar. Making your own desserts is the best way to incorporate more nutrition into desserts and snacks *while reducing the fat and sugar.*

Here are a few examples of foods from each of the food groups:

Grains	Vegetables	Fruits	Dairy	Meat/Beans	Oils	Extras
Cereal	Carrots	Oranges	Non-or low-fat:	Lean Beef	*Butter*	Cookies
Bread	Peas	Bananas	Milk	Chicken	Oils	Cake
Oats	Broccoli	Berries	Yogurt	Fish/Pork	*Mayonnaise*	Pie
Rice	Spinach	Cherries	Cheese	Nuts/seeds	Nuts	Chips
Pasta	Cabbage	Pineapple		Beans/Legumes	Avocado	Candy

Things to be aware of:

- Homemade treats are better for you, but still need to be limited to no more than one serving per day.
- Butter, butter substitutes and oil have about 12 grams of fat per tablespoon. While olive oils and nuts are good for us, we still need to limit them because they add excess calories.

♥ **Health Coach Wisdom:** Try a one week experiment. Make an eating plan for the week. Aim to get *at least* one fresh fruit or vegetable with each meal. Grocery shop and prep the produce when you get home. Wash and chop items for snacks and meals. See how easy it is to grab these healthy foods. *Go to www.lynellross.com for a weekly meal planning sheet and more ideas.*

Measure Portion Sizes to Keep Control of Your Weight

How can I tell what a 3 ounce serving of protein is?

A serving of meat (2-3 ounces) is the size of a deck of cards or the palm of your hand. *One ounce* of meat equals:

- 1 egg
- 1 tablespoon of peanut butter
- ¼ cup of cooked beans or dried split peas
- ½ ounce nuts/seeds

How do I watch my portion sizes? *Learn to eye-ball portions, the size of these equals:*

- 6 dice = 1 ½ ounce of cheese
- A baseball = one cup of dry cereal
- ½ baseball = ½ cup cooked cereal or rice
- Tip of your thumb to the first joint = 1 teaspoon of butter or oil
- 3 teaspoons = 1 tablespoon

How much protein should we be eating per day?

An average person on a 2,000 calorie plan needs about 5 ½ ounces per day. A sedentary woman needs about 44 grams. A sedentary man needs only 56 grams. We should get at least 10% to 35% of your daily calories from protein sources, according to the Institute of Medicine. Most dietitians advise getting protein from a variety of sources. There are 2-3 grams of protein in a slice of bread, 2-3 grams in a serving of green vegetables, 8 grams in a cup of milk, and 7 grams in every ounce of meat.

Excess protein is not good for us and depletes us of minerals such as calcium. Too little protein causes our immune system to weaken. Get in the habit of eating protein with each meal in the proper amounts. This will stabilize your blood sugar, help you feel full and help elevate your mood.

If you have been diagnosed with type 2 diabetes, how do you plan your meals?

Many people with diabetes assume they have to cut satisfying foods from their diet. Not true. Managing diabetes focuses on selecting delicious, nutritious foods that aid in blood sugar control. Eating right is essential to keeping blood sugar levels steady and in a safe range. Foods that are best are minimally processed whole foods that are lower in calories and unhealthy fats and have high amounts of nutrients.

♥ **Health Coach Wisdom:** People with type 2 diabetes are not much different from the rest of us—we all need to eat mindfully. If we eat balanced meals and snacks in correct portion sizes, we will maintain a healthy weight. *Please meet with a Registered Dietician if you have diabetes to learn about how to maximize blood sugar control with correct portions and for meal plans.*

To prevent diabetes, heart disease and maintain healthy weight: Eat small meals and small snacks at almost the same time every day. When snacks contain protein, such as yogurt, nuts, hummus, or eggs the *protein* acts as a blood sugar stabilizer by balancing the carbohydrates and keeping your sugars from spiking. Your breakfasts, lunches, and dinners should contain a balanced combination of protein, carbohydrate, and fat. Fruit is pure carbohydrate and, when eaten alone, can sometimes elevate blood sugar levels, so eat fruit with a protein to stay satisfied.

Be careful of added sugars or artificial sweetener in yogurts. To prevent an unhealthy spike in blood sugars eat plain yogurt and add your own fruit. Stay away from food and drinks that contain artificial sweeteners, as these fool your body and confuse your hormones. They can make you crave more sweets!

Getting a variety of fresh nutrients from real food can help you:

- ♥ Resist colds & relieve arthritis pain
- ♥ Reduce and block migraine headaches
- ♥ Reduce inflammation in your joints, back and neck
- ♥ Reduce plaque in arteries, your bad cholesterol, prevent heart disease
- ♥ Boost your immune system and protects you from certain cancers
- ♥ Reduce heartburn
- ♥ Reduce bone loss and Osteoporosis
- ♥ Calm mood swings and prevent depression
- ♥ Stabilize your blood sugar
- ♥ Reduce asthma

♥ **Health Coach Wisdom:** We need a balance of foods to stay healthy. Nutritionists are not happy about the "Low Carb" craze. It is good to cut back on refined white flour and white sugar products, but whole grain foods are necessary for good health. Nutritious carbohydrates provide the body with energy and fuel for the brain and nervous system. Complex carbohydrates are ideal fuel because they have fiber which helps counter act blood sugar spikes. Know and follow your portion sizes.

The following serving size chart provided by the Dairy Council of California can help you visualize correct portion sizes without using measuring cups and spoons:

Serving-Size Comparison Chart

FOOD	SYMBOL	COMPARISON	SERVING SIZE
Milk + Milk Products			
Cheese (string cheese)		Pointer finger	1½ ounces
Milk and yogurt (glass of milk)		One fist	1 cup
Vegetables			
Cooked carrots		One fist	1 cup
Salad (bowl of salad)		Two fists	2 cups
Fruits			
Apple		One fist	1 medium
Canned peaches		One fist	1 cup
Grains, Breads + Cereals			
Dry cereal (bowl of cereal)		One fist	1 cup
Noodles, rice, oatmeal (bowl of noodles)		Handful	½ cup
Slice of whole wheat bread		Flat hand	1 slice
Meat, Beans + Nuts			
Chicken, beef, fish, pork (chicken breast)		Palm	3 ounces
Peanut butter (spoon of peanut butter)		Thumb	1 tablespoon

The Mediterranean Food Guide Pyramid is Recognized for Health Benefits

While there is not just one Mediterranean diet, Oldways, the Harvard School of Public Health, and the European Office of the World Health Organization's Mediterranean Diet Pyramid continues to be a well-known guide to what is universally recognized as the "gold standard" eating pattern that promotes lifelong good health. Research shows that people from the Mediterranean region have the lowest rates of chronic diseases and the highest life expectancy from this type of eating plan:

- An abundance of food from plant sources, including fruits and vegetables, potatoes, breads and grains, beans, nuts, and seeds
- Minimally processed and locally grown foods with antioxidants
- Olive oil as the principal fat, replacing butter and margarine. *Saturated fat consumed not more than a few times per week*
- Daily consumption of low to moderate amounts of cheese and yogurt (low-fat and non-fat versions may be preferable)
- Fish, twice weekly and poultry, up to 7 eggs per week (including in baking)
- Red meat a few times per month. *Limited to 12 to 16 ounces per month; lean versions.*
- Regular physical activity promotes a healthy weight, fitness and well-being
- Moderate consumption of wine, normally with meals; about one to two glasses per day for men and one glass per day for women. *Wine should be considered optional and avoided when consumption would put the individual or others at risk.*

The results from a landmark PREDIMED study and the Mediterranean Diet: a randomized, primary prevention trial of cardiovascular disease found these results: When people follow the Mediterranean pattern of eating, including olive oil and nuts, primarily walnuts, hazelnuts and almonds reduced the risk of cardiovascular diseases by 30%, and specifically reduced stroke by 49%. The benefits also included a reduction in type 2 diabetes, lower levels of inflammatory markers – linked to atherosclerosis, insulin resistance and type 2 Diabetes, reduced arterial pressure, decreased blood lipids and fasting blood glucose and improvement in the management of metabolic syndrome.

♥ **Health Coach Wisdom:** People who follow a Mediterranean-style diet, high in plant foods and cold-water fish (such as salmon), low in red meat and processed foods can reduce inflammation. This helps your arteries. The fat in the Mediterranean diet, mainly from olive oil, nuts and fish, has anti-inflammatory effects. The antioxidants in fruits and vegetables reduce the oxidation of cholesterol-containing particles within artery walls. Avoid high-fructose corn syrup, which goes straight to the liver, where it causes an increase in triglycerides, a major risk factor for heart disease.

Refined Carbohydrates Cause Inflammation in the Body

Refined carbohydrates are found in anything baked with white flour, such as white bread, rolls, crackers, most baked goods, white rice and cheap cereals. They're made by milling whole grains and removing the bran and germ, the two parts of the grain that contain the most nutrients. According to Joy Bauer, Registered Dietician, refined carbohydrates produce a state of inflammation in the body, causing increases in cytokines and other pro-inflammatory compounds, which makes arthritis worse. Limit foods made with refined grains if you want the best chance of reducing arthritis pain. Switch to healthier whole-grains.

Dr. Andrew Weil, M.D. is a pioneer in the field of integrative medicine, with a healing oriented approach to health care which encompasses body, mind and spirit. To prevent heart disease we must take better care of our arteries. Dr. Weil has created his Anti-Inflammatory Food Pyramid, a food plan to take better care of heart health. *For more information, see the resources at the end of this chapter.*

You Are What You Eat

No matter which pyramid or plate you follow, the idea is to ensure you eat a variety of wholesome and nutritional foods. Protect your health by planning to eat healthful meals and snacks, especially breakfast. Breakfast is the most important meal of the day because your brain needs fuel. Eating activates your metabolism first thing in the morning, causing you to burn calories more efficiently all day long.

Dr. Dean Ornish's Program for Reversing Heart Disease

Dr. Dean Ornish's program is based on the landmark research published in the Journal of the American Medical Association and is the only system scientifically proven to reverse heart disease without drugs or surgery. When I first read Dr. Dean Ornish's Program to reverse Heart disease, what struck me most was this:

In short, this is a program about how to enjoy living, not how to avoid dying–how to relax, not how to be lethargic, how to manage stress, not how to avoid it. How to live in a world more fully, not how to withdraw from it. How to take care of yourself so that you can also give more fully to others. The implications of this research go beyond treating and helping to prevent heart disease. Heart disease represents a rich model for examining the relationship between lifestyle and health.

At the end of Dr. Ornish's yearlong study, most patients reported that their chest pains had virtually disappeared: for 82% of the patients, arterial clogging had reversed. They started to feel better almost immediately and today they feel great. Dr. Ornish's patients are thrilled with their new lives. By the standards of conventional medicine, the impossible has happened.

Dr. Ornish offered documented proof that heart disease can be halted or even reversed by simply changing your lifestyle. Participants in his internationally acclaimed scientific study reduced or discontinued medications; their chest pain diminished or disappeared; they felt more energetic, happy and calm; they lost weight while eating more; and blockages in coronary arteries were actually reversed. "We don't know why we choose to eat things that are harmful, smoke cigarettes, and live a sedentary lifestyle, but perhaps it is because it has not been made clear enough what small changes in behavior will do for us, "says Dr. Dean Ornish.

In a recent statement regarding sensational reports regarding fats, Dr. Ornish had this to say: "*When fat calories were carefully controlled, patients lost 67 percent more body fat than when carbohydrates were controlled. An optimal diet for preventing disease is a whole-foods, plant based diet that is naturally low in animal protein, harmful fats and refined carbohydrates. What that means is little or no red meat; mostly vegetables, fruits, whole grains, legumes and soy products in their natural forms; very few simple and refined carbohydrates such as sugar and while flour; and sufficient "good fats" such as fish oil or flax oil, seeds and nuts. A healthful diet should be low in "bad fats, "meaning trans fats, saturated fats and hydrogenated fats. Finally, we need more quality and less quantity.*"

If you have a family history of heart disease, see the resources at the end of this chapter for more information on Dr. Dean Ornish and Dr. Andrew Weil.

♥ **Health Coach Wisdom:** You can take control of your health and your life. Don't let other people do your thinking for you. Get the facts. Decide what is best for you, and then start with small changes.

How to Maintain or Lose Weight Effortlessly

What is the biggest secret to healthy weight loss?
Never go on a diet again!

Create a healthy lifestyle by understanding healthy eating and how it relates to your emotions. Learn the science behind weight loss and weight maintenance so you will be motivated to eat well. *What you tell yourself about what you eat may be preventing you from losing weight.* Be kind to yourself to reduce stress in your life. Stop torturing yourself about the way you look and start thinking of your weight as a way to be healthy and fit. A realistic, healthy weight will help you to feel good about the way you look and feel.

To lose weight, you must discover *why you are overweight.* Examine emotional reasons for eating. If you are an emotional eater, consider working with a nutritionist, Registered Dietician, therapist or wellness coach, *to get support.* Plan meals, shop for good food, prepare healthy meals, make good choices when eating out and allow yourself to **ENJOY WHAT YOU EAT.**

♥ **Health Coach Wisdom:** Change the way you think about how you eat, by changing the words you use:

➢ Choose **Lifestyle** over diet
➢ Choose **Choice** over cheat
➢ Choose **Good** over bad

The word diet is a noun meaning: "The foods eaten by a particular group." In our culture the word has taken on a negative connotation. Going on a *"diet"* is associated with being hungry, deprived and even starved. American diets usually cut out one or more of the food groups, so people lose weight only because calories are restricted by default. The minute we "go off" the diet we revert back to old habits and we put the weight back on. Are you tired of this? Would you like to learn a better way to lose weight and keep it off naturally?

When you eat nutritious foods, in the correct amounts for your body, you will reach and maintain a healthy weight. I know that sounds too simple, yet feeding your body from the food groups in proper amounts is the key take away message!

First gather a few basic facts about *you.* How much do you currently weigh? How tall are you? How active are you? Then decide on a healthy weight. Get the facts and decide based on your health.

> Understand that self-respect and self-acceptance are the
> cornerstones of permanent health and weight loss.
> ~ Christiane Northrup, M.D.

A healthy weight is a weight that allows you to feel energetic, reduce health risks and improves the quality of your life. *Refer to the Body Mass Index Chart in Chapter one, to find a healthy weight range for your height.* This chart is based on disease risk and does not take into account how fit you are, but it is a good starting point.

Our bodies store fat when it is not used as energy. A calorie is a unit of food energy. How many calories are stored as fat depends on the amount of food you eat and how active you are. Once you accept this, you gain control and make your own choices. You never have to diet again.

You will make choices about *what* you will eat every day and *how much.* You will make choices about how and when *you move your body.* If you follow the recommendations of experts, and listen to your own inner wisdom about what is best for you, a shift will occur. When you remove your emotions and view it as science, you can quickly go from negative thinking to positive thinking, from punishment to reward, from deprivation to appreciation. If you have emotional eating issues, getting support can help, but first arm yourself with information.

♥ **Health Coach Wisdom:** Losing even 5-10% of your weight can significantly improve your health! An overweight or obese, post menopausal woman who loses just 5% of her weight could potentially cut her risk of breast cancer by 50%. The National Cancer Institute advises maintaining a healthy weight to reduce breast cancer risk.

Refer to the following weight chart to find a healthy weight for you:

Height	Weight in Pounds 19-34 years	Weight in pounds > 35 years
5'0"	97-128	108-138
5'1"	101-132	111-143
5'2"	104-137	115-148
5'3"	107-141	119-152
5'4"	111-146	122-157
5'5"	114-150	126-162

Height	Weight in Pounds 19-34 years	Weight in pounds > 35 years
5'6"	118-155	130-167
5'7"	121-160	134-172
5'8"	125-164	138-178
5'9"	129-169	142-183
5'10"	132-174	146-188
5'11"	136-179	151-194
6'0"	140-184	155-199
6'1"	145-189	159-220
6'2"	150-194	164-224

Do you know how many calories you need to just maintain your weight?

There are a variety of ways to estimate the number of calories you need each day to maintain your weight. A simple method is to multiply your weight by a number that represents how active you are. Do you know how many calories you need to maintain your weight? *Most people don't. That is why they gain weight.*

Estimated Daily Requirements: choose your activity level from the chart below then multiple that number by your current weight. _____ X _____ = **the number of calories you need each day to maintain your weight.** If you exercise, you add in the amount of calories you burn. *For example, if you walk at a moderate speed for 30 minutes you will burn approximately 200 calories, depending on how much you weigh. Refer to Chapter 3 for more information on exercise and calorie burning.*

Activity Level	Sedentary/light – little activity	Moderate	Strenuous
Female	12	13	15
Male	13	15	17

Sedentary & Light: walking 3 mph, housecleaning, golf w/cart
Moderate: walking 4mph, cycling, skiing, dancing
Heavy: walking uphill, basketball, running, climbing

Take your current weigh and multiply it by the appropriate activity level number. Example: 150 lb. x 12 = 1800 calories needed to maintain weight for a 150 pound woman who is lightly active. If she adds in a 30 minute walk per day, she increases her calorie needs to 2,000 per day.

You now understand how many daily calories you need to eat per day to maintain your weight. To lose 1 pound, you will need to decrease caloric intake by 3,500 calories—the number of calories it take to gain or lose 1 pound. The easiest way to do this is to cut your calories by 500 per day, so in 7 days you will lose 1 pound.

♥ **Health Coach Wisdom:** *Weight loss is best achieved slowly by losing only 1-2 pounds per week!* If this sounds too slow to you, consider that it took you a long time to put the weight on, and to lose it safely and easily, allow yourself a reasonable amount of time to take it off. You will feel better as soon as you start to make healthier choices, and will not be denying yourself.

The Easiest Way to Lose Weight

For most people, the best way to lose weight is to eat three *appropriate* size meals and two or three *small* nutritious snacks daily instead of skipping then eating large meals.

Your meal plan should provide carbohydrates, fat and protein. The easiest way is to eat from food groups, use "My Plate", or Mediterranean Pyramid as a guide, making sure you eat three balanced meals *around* 300 to 450 calories each and snacks around 150 – 200 calories.

The exact amount depends on your size and weight. Eating balanced meals and snacks helps prevent your blood sugar from crashing and keeps you satisfied. You won't be hungry and you will make better choices. *It is also important to drink water throughout the day.*

After you take the time at the beginning to keep track of what you are eating, you won't have to keep looking things up or logging them. The objective is to develop the habit of eating healthful foods in the proper portions. That is the key to building a healthy lifestyle. Once you master *what* to eat, *how much* to eat and *why* you eat, by listening to your body, you will never have to struggle with a weight problem again.

♥ **Health Coach Wisdom: Keep a Food Log!** The most powerful predictor of weight loss is to accurately track what you eat and drink. If you are serious about wanting to lose weight, buy a notebook and write down everything you eat and drink. Start with two weeks and see what

> changes! *For example, just one ounce of cheese, one slice, has 9 grams of fat and 5 grams of saturated fat. Eating too much cheese is one of the primary sources of weight gain because people do not realize how many calories and fat grams they are truly eating.*

Help Yourself Succeed by Keeping a Food Diary

Researchers at Louisiana State University asked dietitians to estimate their daily caloric intake, *and even the professionals underestimated the number by ten percent.* That may explain why some people don't understand why they are having trouble losing weight. The simple solution: Keep a food diary or track foods online.

When researchers from Kaiser Permanente Center for Health Research followed more than 2,000 people who were encouraged to record meals and snacks, they found that the single best predictor of whether a participant would drop weight was whether the person kept a food diary. The number of pounds people lost was directly related to the number of days they wrote in their log.

The National Diabetes Prevention Program asks participants to keep track of their food intake and exercise minutes for the 16 week core program *and optionally for the next year.* Those that log are the most successful at preventing diabetes, lowering their blood sugar and improving their health numbers.

"My Plate" Method for Weight Loss

If you are resistant to keeping a food log or counting calories yet want to lose weight, then try the "My Plate" method. *Healthful weight loss is about portion size, not excluding food groups.* Divide your plate into 4 sections for each meal. Place protein in one quarter, whole grains in one quarter, fruit in one quarter and vegetables in the last. Add a glass of fat-free milk and/or water. Eat **m-i-n-d-f-u-l-l-y.** If you are still hungry, eat more vegetables or salad. Vegetables are low in calories, high in fiber and nutrition which help you feel full. Have something like a portion of nuts for a snack. *Visit www.supertracker.usda.gov for more information.*

♥ **Health Coach Wisdom:** Eat foods that are nutrient dense, *they deliver the most nutrients for the least amount of calories.* Avoid foods that are *low in nutrient* density, such as potato chips and candy. They are "empty calories" because they are mostly sugar or fat with little or no vitamins or minerals. When eating whole foods, fruits, vegetables, lean means, fat-free or low-fat dairy and whole grains you can eat more volume for a lot less calories than processed "products". *Consider the difference between a scone and vanilla latté at 1,000 calories versus a scrambled egg, whole grain toast, coffee with fat-free milk, and a half cup of sliced strawberries, totaling less than 300 calories with far less fat and sugar.*

Are you Afraid of Being Hungry?

Many people who are overweight are often afraid of feeling hungry, causing them to overeat. Understanding your feelings will help you control your decision to eat. When you cut down on large portions and stop eating "anything you want, anytime you want", you may feel hungry at first. Once you begin eating three smaller meals and two snacks per day, you will identify real hunger versus "the thought" of being hungry. When you skip meals, you sabotage yourself. Remember, you are in control. Respect your body and the food you eat and you will achieve your healthy body weight and maintain it by continuing to make conscious choices. The next time you get the urge to eat, ask yourself, "Is it physical hunger or just a thought?"

Physical Hunger	Appetite Trigger
Happens several hours past a snack or meal	Happens randomly
Builds slowly	Develops suddenly
Goes away after eating a proper amount	Stays with you after eating
Happens in your stomach	Happens in your head as a thought
You feel satisfied after eating	You feel guilt after eating

Stretch beyond your current limits.
We can do just about anything we really want and make up our minds
to do. We are all capable of greater things than we realize.
~ Norman Vincent Peale, author, *The Power of Positive Thinking*

How to Prevent Hunger and Food Cravings

Once you have identified the fear of being hungry, you can help prevent that hungry feeling by learning to stabilize your blood sugar. High blood sugar levels can put your heart health at risk. What's more, people who overeat and stuff their stomachs, often "feel" hungry shortly after eating because their hormones and blood sugar are out of whack. Eating less will actually help you feel better! If you find yourself feeling a little hungry, here are some tips for helping you with that uncomfortable feeling:

- ♥ **Drink a glass of water.** Water immediately takes away that empty feeling.
- ♥ **Stop and get quiet.** Ask yourself if this burning or hunger sensation is coming from your fluctuating hormones.
- ♥ **Check in with yourself.** Have you eaten proper meals and snacks? Did you eat a good breakfast and mid-morning snack? Is it lunch time? If you are eating breakfast, lunch, dinner and snacks to help keep your blood sugar levels balanced, you won't get ravenous.
- ♥ **Being mindful** will prevent you from eating unnecessary calories. Mindfulness is the non-judgmental awareness of what is happening at the present moment. If you are honest with yourself, the "hungry feeling" may pass.

To get a handle on blood sugar, choose foods that your body digests slowly so that blood sugar is then released into your bloodstream slowly and steadily. Here are some of the best foods to help you:

- **Beans** are nutritious, low in fat and high in fiber. High fiber foods slow down digestion. Lentils are especially great for stabilizing blood sugar.
- **Whole grains:** (Good carbohydrates) Not only do whole grains digest more slowly than refined, white flour, 100% whole grains keep your blood sugar steady and they are packed with nutrients and fiber.
- **Fresh Fruits and Vegetables**: Low in calories, high in fiber, rich in anti-inflammatory antioxidants and tasty, fresh produce makes them the perfect food for stabilizing blood sugar levels.
- **Fish:** This lean protein provides omega-3 fatty acids to protect your heart.
- **Fat-free or low-fat dairy:** Another good choice for lean protein.
- **Nuts:** Nuts fill you up with fiber and omega-3 fatty acids and satisfy that need for something crunchy. Eat the proper portion size, which is a ¼ cup serving.

365,000 people die each year from obesity related diseases! To reduce your waistline, stabilize your blood sugar, and assure better health, eat these foods *sparingly*. (*Notice I didn't say eliminate, unless you want to. The key to building healthy habits is to allow yourself treats or you won't want to continue. You will make better choices when you think about how you affect your health with what you eat*):

- **Refined grains:** White breads, white pasta, white rice and refined flours all get digested quickly by the body, sending your blood sugar on a roller-coaster ride. Switch to whole grains as much as possible. Refined grains such as white flour are devoid of nutrients. *Whole grains have fiber which promotes healthy digestion and prevents constipation. Fiber also helps reduce the unhealthy cholesterol in your blood and helps keep blood sugar levels from spiking, which helps prevent heart disease.*
- **Sugary foods and beverages like soda:** Sugar is digested quickly, flooding your bloodstream with glucose. Consuming too much sugar causes health related problems such as obesity, inflammation, heart disease and more. *You do not have to give up added sugars completely—* ***just eat them sparingly***.
- **Red meat:** *Cutting back* on meat will help you reduce your intake of saturated fat, the bad-for-your-heart kind. Choose lean cuts and be careful to trim visible fat, drain off grease.
- **Fried foods:** French fries, onion rings, deep fried fish, donuts and other fried foods (like fried appetizers) are another source of saturated fat to avoid. **They are loaded with calories, a**ffecting both weight gain and blood sugar. Worse, because of the high heat associated with the oil, fried foods are linked with possible cancers.

Eating too much of any food—even healthful foods—is bad for your body. When you take in more calories than you need, your body gets more of everything than it can handle, throwing your blood sugar and hormones out of balance.

> According to the Mayo clinic, *"Your weight is a balancing act, and calories are part of that equation. Fad diets may promise you that counting carbohydrates or eating a mountain of grapefruit will make the pounds drop off. But when it comes to weight loss, it's calories that count. Weight loss comes down to burning more calories that you take in. You can do that by reducing extra calories from food and beverages and increasing calories burned through physical activity."*

♥ **Health Coach Wisdom: DO NOT DROP CALORIE CONSUMPTION BELOW 1200 per day.** *A big mistake people make when trying to lose weight is actually eating too little.* Remember, *this is not a diet*, it is a lifestyle. When you starve yourself, your metabolism slows down and your body hangs onto your fat for reserve. The best things you can do are to eat within your range, give your body wholesome nutrients and move to recharge your metabolism!

To Help People Lose Weight, The National Diabetes Prevention Program Teaches Participants to Aim For These Ranges:

Your Current Weight LBS	Calorie Range	Fat Gram Range
120-170	1200-1500	33-40
175-215	1500-1800	42-50
220-245	1800-2000	50-60
250-300	2000-2200	55-66

Please note: these are just ranges. Don't obsess about each calorie and fat gram. Simply keep track and stay *near* your range or eat by measuring portion size.

Reading Food Labels 101

How do you know what is in your food? Do you know how many calories, fat grams, or how much fiber and sodium you are getting? The best way to protect yourself from making mistakes is to be informed about the foods you eat by learning to read food labels properly. Refer to the label provided by the Dairy Council of California:

Look at the number of calories and the number of servings. At a glance, the label on that soda or tea might say 100 calories. **Now look at the serving size**: 2.5 servings. The total number of calories in that drink just jumped to 250. The sugar is probably equivalent to 16 teaspoons.

Look at the ingredients. Don't be fooled. The ingredients on the label of all prepared foods lists each ingredient by the largest amount included first, the next most prominent second and so on in descending order. When buying cereal for example, it is good if the grain is listed first, but if high fructose corn syrup or sugar is listed first, it contains more sugar than anything else.

Watch out for dyes, MSG, trans-fats, artificial and other unwanted ingredients that can cause headaches, fatigue and even cancers. For more information on ingredients to avoid visit my website at www.lynellross.com.

Nutrition Facts

Serving Size 8 fl oz (245g)
Servings Per Container 8

Amount Per Serving

Calories 170   Calories from Fat 20

%Daily Value*

	%Daily Value*
Total Fat 2.5g	4 %
Saturated Fat 1.5g	8 %
Trans Fat 0g	0 %
Cholesterol 5mg	2 %
Sodium 190mg	8 %
Total Carbohydrate 29g	10 %
Dietary Fiber 1g	5 %
Sugars 27g	
Protein 8g	

Vitamin A 10%	•	Vitamin C	6%
Calcium 30%	•	Iron	4%

* Percent Daily Values are based on a 2,000 calorie diet.

Check the label for sugar grams: Sugar isn't always *added* to foods, some have natural sugar. Here is a quick way to determine the number of teaspoons of sugar: Divide the number of grams of sugar by 4 to get the number of teaspoons of sugar. One teaspoon of granulated sugar has 4 grams. If a container of yogurt has 16 grams of sugar–that is roughly 4 teaspoons of sugar. **Percent Daily Value:** This tells the percentage of the recommended daily amount of each nutrient in one serving of a food. Labels are based on a 2,000 calorie diet.

Understand Fats: Limit your intake of saturated fats and sodium to 5 percent or less per serving of food. Beware of trans-fats, the harmful fat that raises your bad cholesterol (LDL) and lowers your good cholesterol (HDL). *Aim for ZERO Trans fats.*

❤ **Health Coach Wisdom:** Buy a book such as *Calorie King, Calorie, Fat & Carbohydrate Counter* that lists calories, fat grams and carbohydrates in food. Or search on-line at websites such as www. myfitnesspal.com. You will find more resource listings at the end of this chapter for great websites that will give you food and nutrient values and even keep track of your totals. It is easy. The program does all the work.

How Fat Can Help or Hurt You

We need fat to survive, although most of us eat too much fat. A necessary nutrient with positive health benefits, fat helps us feel full longer. Fats work with other nutrients that are carried into our blood stream to nourish our bodies. However, a high fat diet, especially one high in animal fat, can lead to heart disease, cancer, diabetes and obesity. The key is in knowing about the types of fat as well as the amounts our bodies need.

Focus on good fats: monounsaturated fats in olive oil, canola oil, nuts and avocados, polyunsaturated fats in omega-3's in fish, flax meal, walnuts, and seeds to balance out our needs. Unhealthy fats such as saturated fat, found in butter and cream comes primarily from animal fat. *Saturated fats in excess and hydrogenated fats have been shown to increase cholesterol and heart disease.* The chemical process that converts vegetable oil into margarine also creates trans–fats, which turn out to be worse for your cholesterol than the saturated fat in butter. Fats are higher in calories than other foods, so when you eat less fat, you control your weight more easily.

How Fat Can Prevent You from Maintaining Your Weight

- Fatty foods can seem addicting—but you can break the cycle. Crunchy French fries, pastries, creamy milkshakes and juicy burgers hit your taste buds and leave you wanting more. *Make smarter choices to re-boot your taste buds.*
- Eating too much fat, especially saturated fat and trans-fat, is linked to higher blood cholesterol and a greater risk of diseases.
- Trans-fatty acids formed during the process of partial hydrogenation, act as saturated fats and raise blood cholesterol levels and contribute to heart disease. Avoid products which list hydrogenated oils on the label, these include packaged donuts, pastries, cookies, crackers, cake mixes and snacks.
- Every gram of fat has 9 calories, *twice the amount of carbohydrate or protein.*

♥ **Health Coach Wisdom:** A package may say trans-fat free, however, one serving may still contain .5g. If you eat more than one serving, you could eat as much as 1 to 2 grams or more of dangerous trans-fats. *Beware and read food labels.*

Here are a few ways to cut back on unhealthy fats:

Instead of this:	Substitute a better choice:
Whole milk or cream	Fat-free or 1%milk, soy milk, almond milk
Cheddar or Jack Cheese	Part skim mozzarella, low-fat cottage, parmesan cheese
Butter	Olive oil, Canola oil, buttery spreads such as Smart Balance or Earth Balance
Sour Cream	Low-fat or fat-free sour cream or yogurts
Ground beef or sausage	Lean ground turkey, chicken or soy protein
Store bought cookies, cakes pie, muffins	Homemade cookies, bars, muffins, fruit crumbles
Doughnuts or pastries	Whole grain breads, homemade muffins
Candy bars	Walnuts, almonds and other nuts, dark chocolate

Eat food. Not too much. Mostly plants.
~Michael Pollan, *Food Rules*

Getting Started with Weight Loss

Focus on the positive. The power of positive eating is in concentrating on foods that are good for you. Eat sensibly, getting back to basics like vegetables, fruits and whole grains, lean proteins, and non-fat or low-fat dairy. The healthiest way to live is to incorporate fitness into your routine, while enjoying delicious, healthful foods. Don't fool yourself. For the first week or two, record everything you eat. Studies have proven that keeping a food diary with a detailed account of what you eat and drink results in double the success rate as those who don't keep a journal. Keeping track of everything you eat and drink will help understand why you make certain choices and will reveal your habits. Learn about mindful eating to help you slow down and be aware of what you put in your body.

Use affirmations throughout the day to help you change the way you think. Research shows that affirmations are effective tools for changing the way people think and behave. Instead of being mad at yourself, change your thought to:

I love my body and I take care of it.

Instead of thinking that you can't control your eating, repeat the affirmation:

I choose healthy foods to nourish my body.

Don't tell yourself that *you have been bad* or that a food is *bad* or that you can't have a certain food. Make your choices based on what you know is nourishing for your body. Choose foods from the food groups, allowing for *some* "discretionary" calories, or treats. Make conscious choices. It is empowering to think of the foods you eat as nourishing your body and making you stronger. Think of food in a positive way. Prepare delicious things to eat and when dining out select nutritious dishes.

Are You Stuck? Weight Loss Strategies:

If you have tried losing weight or getting in shape in the past only to fall back into unhealthy habits, here are some tips that will help you overcome your self-sabotaging behaviors and win the prize of a healthy lifestyle:

Be realistic about your healthy weight. If you select a weight based on a number you once were, it may not be realistic. To get off the diet roller coaster, choose a weight that works for you, at the age you are now. Focus on getting healthy and strong.

Be patient. It takes time to lose weight, even up to a year or more if you have 100 pounds or more to lose. It takes time to gain the weight, so being patient. *Safe, lasting weight loss should occur at the rate of about of 1-2 pounds per week.*

Eat a healthy breakfast. Breakfast eaters are slimmer than breakfast skippers who are more than four times more likely to be obese. Research over the past thirty years has shown without fail that breakfast is a key factor in weight control. Your body slows down when you sleep and doesn't speed up until you put fuel in it again. *Donuts and white flour sugary pastries are not good choices.* Breakfast with protein, such as eggs or egg whites with veggies or oatmeal with walnuts help with weight management, blood sugar and mood! *What's more, studies published in the American Heart Association journal showed that those who skipped breakfast had a higher risk of heart attack.*

♥ **Health Coach Wisdom:** Don't exercise first thing in the morning on an empty stomach. After sleeping, about 70% of your glycogen storage is depleted. Nutritionists know fat burns in a carbohydrate flame. You need good carbohydrates to help break down and burn your stored fats. Eating even a small snack can ignite your fat burning metabolism.

Get enough sleep. Regulatory hormones are secreted during sleep. Lack of sleep could possibly affect the proper sequence of hormone release. Staying up late, eating and drinking, will sabotage weight loss efforts.

Watch your stress. Stress can lead to weight gain in people who manage their feelings with food, eating mindlessly, and perceiving food as a soothing friend. Don't blame yourself for gaining weight. It has happened over time while portions have gotten larger and we have become more sedentary. You can make changes now.

Do not skip meals. Skipping meals leads to food cravings and overeating later in the day. When you skip meals and snacks, your metabolism shuts down and alters its calorie-burning abilities and begins to store fat.

Be mindful of calories. Most people think they are cutting back on **portions**, but may not realize the real number of calories they are eating. Use measuring utensils.

Don't sabotage success on the weekends. If you are mindful all week, only to over indulge on the weekend, this may be a clue for why you are not losing weight. It doesn't take much to undo the success you've had.

Focus on the positive. The power of positive eating means concentrating on foods that are good for you. Find nutritious foods you enjoy.

Eat mindfully. Think before you eat. Develop an eating pattern you can live with that is healthful and enjoyable. Don't deny yourself anything, because you will crave that certain food even more. If you want a treat, allow yourself the correct portion size and count it in your daily total of servings. Sit down, concentrate on what you are eating and be appreciative. *This works!!!*

Calorie Counts in Alcoholic Beverages Add Up

One of the reasons for excess weight is that we don't count the calories in our beverages. Remember, everything counts. Another mistake is eating well all week, only to *forget about healthy eating and drinking habits on the weekend.* You do not have to give up drinking alcoholic beverages or fruit juice. However, you must count your drink calories. Be aware of the sugar in beverages that you mix with alcohol. Consuming too much alcohol makes weight loss difficult as it is quickly stored as excess fat. Alcohol *increases your appetite while reducing inhibitions, so you end up eating more of the wrong foods.* If you enjoy alcoholic beverages, moderation is the key: One five-ounce glass of wine, one 12-ounce beer, or 1½ ounce hard liquor per day.

This table estimates caloric counts from various alcoholic beverages. Each shows a sample serving size. Beware of higher alcohol content (higher percent alcohol or higher proof) and mixing alcohol with other beverages, such as soda, tonic water, fruit juice, or cream as they **increase the calories.**

- *Alcoholic beverages supply empty calories, not essential nutrients.*

Beverage	Example Serving Volume	Approximate Total **Calories**
Beer (regular)	12 oz	150
Beer (light)	12 oz	108
White wine	5 oz	100
Red wine	5 oz	105

Beverage	Example Serving Volume	Approximate Total **Calories**
Sweet dessert wine	3 oz	141
80 proof distilled spirits (gin, rum, vodka, whiskey)	1.5 oz	96

If you don't want to give up alcohol, try these tips:

- Order a wine spritzer (wine and sparkling water) to reduce calories
- Drink light beer
- Avoid sweet drinks like margaritas and rum punch which can contain as many as 500– 800 calories per large cocktail.

♥ **Health Coach Wisdom:** Binge drinking destroys brain cells, affecting you for the rest of your life and sometimes causes death. Other effects can include brain damage, liver damage, kidney damage and heart problems.

Uncover the Clues to Why You Overeat

It is helpful to determine why you are overweight before starting a weight loss program. Once you discover what is causing you to be overweight, you can take control and start making changes. There is a solution to every problem. Let's find out what yours is. Take a few minutes to answer the following questions. *Be honest with yourself* and think carefully. You will discover your troubled areas and make changes that will enable you to live happily at a healthy weight:

Why do *you think* you are overweight? List your ideas_____
_____

Do you eat breakfast? _____ If not why?_____

Do you skip breakfast and/or lunch only to eat most calories in the evening? _____
Do you start "grazing" while you are cooking? _____

Do you eat while you are cleaning up the dishes? _____

Do you believe you are overweight as a result of your eating habits or more because of emotional eating? Why_____
_____

Do have a realistic idea of what your healthy weight is? _____

How does your family history play a part in the kinds of foods you choose and how much that your eat? _____

Are you afraid to lose weight because the change in your appearance may affect someone close to you or for another reason? _____

Do you eat when you are bored? _____ Do you eat more when you are around others because you don't want to hurt their feelings? _____

Do you eat when you are unhappy, angry, anxious, lonely, bored, frustrated or feeling down? _____. *Circle all that apply.*

Do you mainly eat meals and snacks or prepare meals at home?_____

Do you eat when you "think" you are hungry? _____When?_____

Do you binge eat? _____ If so, when? _____

Do you *know* the correct portion sizes for meals and snacks? _____

Write down any clues you uncover relating to your mood and what causes you to lose control or become anxious. Your secret weapon is your food journal and learning to understand any underlying anxiety that may cause you to overeat.

♥ **Health Coach Wisdom:** If you know you are an emotional eater, seek the help of a Registered Dietitian or Therapist. Talking with someone you trust will help uncover reasons you might not be consciously aware of. The support will help you change your thoughts about food and eating. Or try *The Tapping Solution and mindful eating courses* listed at the end of the chapter.

---

10 Secrets for Healthy Eating Out

1. Make a plan of what to order and have a snack before your meal.
2. Choose low-fat foods that are baked or grilled.
3. Enjoy iced tea, sparkling water or coffee while waiting for your meal.
4. Control portion sizes by asking for a container with your meal. Then package it up and put it aside.
5. Eat slowly and pay attention to your food and the person you are dining with.
6. Begin your meal with a salad or soup (without a cream base).
7. Ask for vegetables as your side dish instead of fries.
8. Order sauces and dressings on the side so you control the amount you eat.
9. Share an entrée with someone else. You'll save money too!
10. Go online to review calorie and nutrition counts of your favorite restaurants. You will be surprised at the high calorie and fat content.

Keeping a food journal is the most powerful tool you can use for weight loss and behavior change. Recording your eating and exercise habits provides a revealing account of what you eat, drink and how much you move. Notice how many servings you get from each food group. What are you missing?

Ready to get started? Make copies of My Daily Record to log your food and beverages!

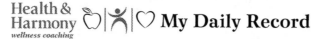 **My Daily Record**

Time of Day	Portion Size or Amount	Description of Food Eaten: *Keep track of which food group: Veggie, fruit, grain, protein, etc.*	*Food Group	Calories	Fat Gram

Totals: _____

*Food Groups: Vegetable, Fruit, (Meat/Bean/Nut/Seed/Legume), Grain, Dairy

Minutes and type of Physical Activity Today: _____

Glasses of Water Today: ❑ ❑ ❑ ❑ ❑ ❑ ❑ ❑ ❑ ❑ ❑ ❑

Aim for eight (eight ounce) glass of water -more if you are active or are in a hot climate.

My moods today were: _____

Visit www.lynellross.com for a downloadable version of this food log.

What's Next For You?

A good health coach will always ask you about your next step. Do you need to pack more powerful nutrition into your day? Do you want to lose weight? Do you need to help improve your cholesterol or blood pressure? Would you like to see a Registered Dietitian? Do you want to learn more about the benefits of eating nutritious foods?

Use your Action Plan to set a goal for your nutrition.

My intention is: _____by this date _____.

The steps I will take to get started are:

1. _____
2. _____
3. _____
4. _____
5. _____

There is no right or wrong way to eat.
~Dr. Jan Chozen Bays, Author of *Mindful Eating*

For more on healthy eating, go to these resources for nutrition and health:

Academy of Nutrition and Dietetics, www.eatright.org

Food and Nutrition information you can trust. It's all about eating right. Registered dietitians are food and nutrition experts, translating the science of nutrition into practical solutions.

American Heart Association, www.americanheart.org. *Resources for managing heart health, stroke and heart attack prevention.*

Center for Science in the Public Interest, www.cspinet.org. *Sign up for the Nutrition Action Healthletter. It is the most reliable source you can find, packed with unbiased information on nutrition, health, food products, restaurants and recipes.*

The Ornish Spectrum, www.ornishspectrum.com, a proven program that heals hearts and transforms lives, information about how you can prevent and reverse heart disease with Dr. Ornish's 37 years of scientifically proven integrative lifestyle program. *You can improve chronic conditions such as heart disease, diabetes and cancers.*

Centers for Disease Control and Prevention, www.cdc.gov

National Institutes of Health, www.nih.gov

USDA, www.choosemyplate.gov, tips on healthy eating, meal planning and nutrition

Fruits and Veggies More Matters. www.fruitsandveggiesmorematters.org. *Healthy eating tips, meal plans, shopping tips, recipes and suggestions for eating 5- 9 servings of fruits and vegetables daily.*

California Dairy Council, www.healthyeating.org, information, nutrition, meal planning and workplace wellness tips. www.nationaldairycouncil.org. www.mealsmatter.

Nutrition Center at the Mayo Clinic, www.mayohealth.org

Everyday Health, www.everydayhealth.com, *Calorie counter, meal planner and health information.*

Spark People, www.sparkpeople.com, *calorie tracker, recipes, information and more.*

CalorieKing, www.calorieking.com, *weight loss tips, calorie tracker and support*

My Fitness Pal, www.myfitnesspal.com, calorie and nutrition tracking online and more.

The Tapping Solution by Nick Ortner, and *The Tapping Solution for Weight Loss and Body Confidence* by Jessica Ortner. www.thetappingsolution.com., help with emotional eating.

Dr. Andrew Weil, www.drweil.com.*for health information, serving sizes and a printable download of Dr. Weil's pyramid, books and resources.*

Mediterranean Diet & Pyramid, www.oldwayspt.org. The "gold standard" eating pattern that promotes lifelong good health. Download a PDF of the pyramid.

The Center for Mindful Eating, www.thecenterformindfuleating.org/jan-chozen-bays. The author of *Mindful Eating*, Jan Chozen Bays teaches courses on mindful eating which leads to better eating habits.

For more information on weight loss, health eating tips, emotional eating, recipes meal planning and wellness coaching, go to my website: www.lynellross.com.

Chapter 3

Fit Fitness into Your Day

Exercise is the closest thing we'll ever get to the miracle pill that everyone
is seeking. It brings weight loss, appetite control, improved mood and self-
esteem, an energy kick, and longer life by decreasing the risk of heart
disease, diabetes, stroke, osteoporosis, and chronic disabilities.
~Werner W.K. Hoeger and Sharon A. Hoeger,
Principles and Labs for Fitness and Wellness

What is the Number One Reason People Cite for Not Exercising?

Lack of time is the number one reason given for not exercising. Only *you* can decide if this is really true for you. It sounds reasonable, but ask yourself: *Is it really a lack of time or would you rather do anything else but exercise?* We are busy with work, children, laundry, cleaning, paying bills, yard work and helping relatives in our daily lives. Of course, we can't find a minute to exercise. When we do find time, we are too exhausted to move. Does this sound familiar?

If you are discouraged about your lack of exercise, there is hope for you. Research has proven that *if you find your own inner motivation* you will make time to be active and exercise. But how do you find your motivation? To start, question the way you think about exercise. You can always find time to do things you want to do. *Exercise does not have to mean hours of sweating at the gym.* The old way of thinking that you have to lift heavy weights or subject yourself to hours of "no pain-no gain" exercises are over. You can begin to make positive changes in as little as ten minutes a day. When you begin to move, endorphins kick in and you feel better.

Research indicates that Americans need only do thirty minutes or more daily of moderate activity, such as walking, for *health benefits*. Exercise can help you prevent or manage heart disease, diabetes, arthritis, Alzheimer's, cancer, menopause, osteoporosis, back pain and more! You can break up those thirty minutes into ten minute segments throughout the day. If the idea of finding time for thirty minutes to exercise exhausts you, consider this: There are twenty-four hours in each day. If you aim for eight hours of sleep, that leaves sixteen hours. No matter what responsibilities you have, *if you can't find a couple of ten minute segments to take a time out for yourself to go for a walk or stretch break, then you will burn out and your health will suffer. You can begin with just ten minutes.*

♥ **Health Coach Wisdom:** If you wait for a special time to be active, it may not happen. Take five or ten minutes *throughout your day.* Gently stretch before you take your shower in the morning. Walk for twenty minutes during your lunch break. Take the stairs. Do push-ups at your kitchen counter. Do a few squats and crunches while you watch TV in the evening to automatically fit fitness into your day. Take short walks throughout your day for an energy boost that will invigorate your body and mind. Everything counts. Connecting to a few minutes of movement keeps you in the habit of exercising.

Whatever your age make good health rather than good looks your motivation for getting fit.
~ Susan McQuinllan, M.S., R.D.N

Exercise should not be a chore or something to fear. Done properly, it can be a break for you, a time to stretch, relieve back pain, to "walk off" a stressful day and get some quiet time. Your attitude about exercise is everything. If you think of it as something *you get to do*, you will want to exercise. If you have had a bad experience with exercise in the past, then it is time to reconsider what happened. You *should start slowly, go at your own pace and take it easy. Do something that feels good.*

Here are some common objections to exercise with *some possible solutions:*

♥ I don't like to sweat. *You get to decide at what level of intensity to exercise, but do you know sweating is good for you? It releases toxins and clears your skin among other benefits. Moving enough to sweat means you are helping your heart get stronger.*

♥ I don't want to go to the gym where people will judge me. *There are some great fitness centers such as Curves and Anytime Fitness where you can go at your own pace.*

♥ I don't want to be seen in a swimsuit so I won't take a water aerobics class. *You can wear a T shirt, or cover up in the water. The other participants are self-conscious and not judging you. Most water classes are supportive and really fun!*

♥ My knees or back hurts. *Ride a recumbent bike or water walk to take pressure off.*

♥ It hurts to exercise and I feel out of breath. *Think of the benefits while taking time to work up to a moderate level of intensity. Start slowly and be gentle with yourself.*

While these are understandable objections, you can find a solution to every exercise dilemma. If you feel out of breath and it doesn't feel good to exercise it may be that you are out of condition. You must be patient. It will take time to get back into shape. It is best to build up slowly over time. Every bit of movement helps you burn calories so you can lose weight, and best of all, exercising makes you feel great, vibrant and alive! It builds your self-esteem. *Everything you do counts!* You can start by walking and moving around more during the day.

♥ **Health Coach Wisdom:** Today, head out of your door and walk for five minutes; then walk back. That is your ten minute segment. Do this three times a week and then increase to twenty minutes. You will be stronger and feel great about yourself. It is that simple and more beneficial than you know.

> You will never change your life until you change something you do daily. The secret of your success is found in your daily routine.
> ~ John C. Maxwell

If you do not have a regular exercise program, you may not have experienced the benefits of exercise. If you take one thing away from this chapter, I hope it is that you will begin to see *exercise as movement that makes you feel good*. You do not have to participate in an exercise class to reap the benefits from moving. Exercise also comes in the form of walking, playing tennis, swimming, biking, hiking, washing windows and doing housework. *The important thing is to be aware of the benefits of moving.* Walking will lower your blood pressure and ease stress. The more you move the better you will feel.

How to Fit Fitness Into Your Day

> Not exercising is a depressant.
> ~Tal David Ben-Shahar, Professor of Positive
> Psychology, Harvard University.

- ♥ Meet your friends to walk and talk
- ♥ Take the stairs—this is a great way to raise your heart rate
- ♥ Take your kids or dog for a daily walk
- ♥ Make a habit of getting up for 5 minutes out of every 55 you sit and walk around the building. This helps prevent Type 2 diabetes!

- Do wall or counter push-ups while waiting for your lunch to heat up
- Lift hand weights for 10 minutes while watching TV
- Take a class in dance, yoga or Zumba and keep your weekly date

How Exercise Benefits You

Exercise keeps you moving, healthy and energized. It benefits your mind, body and spirit. Exercise:

- Helps you to stay strong and tone your muscles
- Helps you to sleep better
- Helps reduce stress
- Prevents weight gain, keeps you fit and looking vibrant
- Reduces the risk of falls, injuries and broken bones
- Improves your mood, self-confidence and feelings of self-worth
- Lowers your risk of illness such as heart disease, diabetes and cancer
- Keeps your brain and memory functioning well
- Keeps you independent and able to take care of yourself as you age
- Balances your hormones to keep you happy and much more

How to Embrace Exercise as Part of Your Daily Life

Recent studies have shown that sitting for most of the day increases
the risk of heart disease to a degree similar to that of smoking
~*Mayo Clinic Essential Heart Guide*

With a little planning and by starting slowly, you can make it easy to develop the habit of being active. You will find the benefits *far outweigh the effort*. These tips will help:

Talk to your doctor. Make sure it's safe for you to start an exercise routine or walking program. Learn which exercises are best for you.

Get equipped. You'll need sturdy, supportive shoes for whatever exercise you choose, whether it's walking or biking. Make sure you have comfortable clothing.

Make the time. Set aside time every day for exercise, *or fit it in through your day.* Start by taking the stairs instead of the elevator, or with a walk around the block. Gradually work your way up to longer blocks of time most days of the week. Park farther away from the store and think of it as an opportunity to fit in exercise!

Turn chores into exercise. You don't have to hit the gym for it to count as exercise. Clean your house, mow the lawn, or tackle projects like cleaning out clutter.

Get support. Consider getting a workout buddy to keep you on track or hiring a *qualified, certified* personal trainer to develop a program. A trainer will encourage you to stick with it and help you chart your progress. Hang around people who are fit to inspire you to keep going.

Make it fun. Exercise doesn't have to be an exhausting, sweaty chore that you dread. Enjoy your workout! Go dancing, swimming or bike with your friends.

You'll be amazed at how easy it is to add in small bits of exercise each day and how you'll come to enjoy it. If you want to stay healthy and independent, being active is the key. Remember to eat well before and after exercise. Your body needs fuel to perform.

Exercising Helps Fight Illness

How would you like to escape from getting a cold or the flu this year? You can by exercising regularly. Exercise bolsters the immune system to fight off illness. According to the BBC news, a study of 1,000 people found that staying active reduced catching a cold virus by nearly half and those that did had less severe symptoms. The participants in this study walked or did exercise for 20 minutes five or more days per week. Lifestyle plays a part in reducing colds by as much as 50% for those who are active and eat well.

The Beauty Benefits of Exercise

Exercising not only helps burn calories, aids in weight loss and helps you feel better; it also improves your complexion. Exercise is a great remedy for acne, wrinkles, dull skin and more. When you get your heart pumping from aerobic exercise, you're supplying your skin with a dose of oxygenated blood, giving you a vibrant glow. Exercise helps prevent wrinkles and sagging skin by boosting the production of collagen. The improved blood flow also keeps your hair stronger and healthier, stimulates the hair follicles and promotes growth. Walking, stretching and yoga will improve circulation and reduce stress. Exercising changes the shape of your body by toning your muscles, improving your posture and giving you a lean and healthy look. *This is beauty from the inside out.*

THE FIRST STEP: Before you begin an exercise program, take a fitness test, or substantially increase your level of activity, please answer a few questions. This physical activity readiness questionnaire (PAR-Q) will help determine if you're ready to begin an exercise program.

- Has your doctor ever said that you have a heart condition or that you should participate in physical activity only as recommended by a doctor?
- Do you feel pain in your chest during physical activity?
- In the past month, have you had chest pain when *you were not* doing physical activity?
- Do you lose your balance from dizziness? Do you ever lose consciousness?
- Do you have a bone or joint problem that could be made worse by a change in your physical activity?
- Is your doctor currently prescribing drugs for your blood pressure or a heart condition?
- Do you know of any reason you should not participate in physical activity?

If you answered yes to one or more questions, if you are over 40 years of age and have recently been inactive, or if you are concerned about your health, consult a physician before taking a fitness test or substantially increasing your physical activity.

PRIOR TO EXERCISE

Prior to beginning any exercise program, seek medical evaluation and clearance to engage in activity. Not all exercise programs are suitable for everyone, and some programs may result in injury. Activities should be carried out at a pace that is comfortable for you. Discontinue participation in any exercise activity that causes pain or discomfort. In such event, medical consultation should be immediately obtained.

What Does it Mean to be Physically Fit?

In general, being fit refers to cardiovascular fitness, or how effectively the heart and lungs supply oxygen to the muscles. While it allows you to exercise for a longer period of time or run to catch your dog without getting winded, its most important benefit is a reduced risk of major diseases such as coronary heart disease and stroke.

There are four types of physical fitness:

1. Cardiovascular or Cardiorespiratory
2. Strength Training
3. Flexibility
4. Body Composition

How Much Do I Have to Exercise?

A well rounded physical activity program includes aerobic or cardio exercise, strength training and flexibility. Each of these has specific benefits. While being active for thirty minutes a day provides us with health benefits to help fight off chronic illness, if you participate in all three types of fitness, you will be stronger, healthier and feel better.

The American College of Sports Medicine's physical activity recommendations for healthy adults is at least thirty minutes of moderate-intensity physical activity, working hard enough to break a sweat, but still able to carry on a conversation, five days a week—or do twenty minutes or more of vigorous activity three days a week.

If you are just starting an exercise program, please start slowly and don't push yourself. If you hurt yourself or don't like it, you won't continue. So keep it simple with something like walking short distances or exercising for five or ten minutes at a time. However, if you have been doing the same types of exercise for a while and are in a rut, why set the bar low when you can achieve a state of optimal fitness? Challenge yourself to increase your fitness level. In this chapter we examine the benefits and ways you can incorporate the types of fitness into your life.

What is Cardiorespiratory Fitness?

Cardiorespiratory Fitness describes the health and function of the heart, lungs and circulatory system. It is related to endurance, or the ability to sustain activity for prolonged periods. It is also known as aerobic exercise, and can be achieved with such activities as walking briskly, going uphill, running, biking or swimming. Raising your heart rate strengthens your heart muscle. Other aerobic activities include stair climbing, rowing and cross country skiing.

Cardio fitness also describes the capacity of the lungs to exchange oxygen and carbon dioxide with the blood and the circulatory system's ability to transport blood and nutrients to tissues for sustained periods without undue fatigue. Cardiovascular health goes beyond aerobic fitness. It defines the status of the heart muscle, its blood vessels and the circulatory system. *Cardiorespiratory fitness means you have a strong heart!*

♥ **Health Coach Wisdom:** The most important thing on my "To Do" list is getting some type of cardio exercise at least four days per week to help me prevent heart disease.

If you are not physically fit right now, be patient. You can begin by walking ten minutes at a time. You receive benefits by *accumulating* thirty minutes of exercise most days of the week. Walk in sets of ten minutes throughout the day. To test your fitness, see how fast you can walk a mile without getting winded. It should take no more than eighteen minutes for moderately fit women in their thirties or forties. Subtract thirty seconds less for men. For those past age forty, allow an extra 30 seconds for each additional decade.

Here are a few good reasons to get moving:

The Benefits of Cardiorespiratory Fitness Include:

- ♥ Reduction in blood pressure
- ♥ Increase in the HDL or "healthy" cholesterol
- ♥ Decreased body fat stores—*Helping you burn body fat*
- ♥ Increased aerobic capacity—*Increase in maximal oxygen consumption*
- ♥ Decreased symptoms of anxiety, tension and depression
- ♥ Helps balance your blood sugar and prevent type 2 diabetes
- ♥ Increased heart function and improved blood flow to blood vessels.
- ♥ Decreases the risk of cardiovascular disease, heart attacks and stroke.
- ♥ Reduction in deaths of patients after heart attack

♥ **Health Coach Wisdom:** Every movement we make involves our muscular system. That means every time you move, from getting up out of your chair to walking up stairs, you are using your muscles. This helps keep you strong and fit, preventing injury among other benefits. You become stronger with every bit of activity you do. Move as much as you can.

The Easiest Way to Become Fit: *Walking For Fitness & Health*

I have not always been in the field of health and fitness. When I was in my forties, I wasn't fit at all. When our children were young, our family went on a vacation with friends. One Sunday, we were at a park having a picnic when the kids organized a soccer game with the kids versus the parents. After a few minutes I was out of breath, could not run and was completely exhausted. I wasn't quite sure what to do about it. I had a belief that mothers just got out of shape because they were too busy to take care of themselves.

A few weeks later, I had a check- up with a caring female doctor who asked me if I was exercising. I replied that I was not. She asked me if I would walk for ten minutes one day per week. I said yes, and the next day I went for my ten minute walk. Her suggestion started me moving again. For a couple of years I walked a few times a week for twenty minutes and then increased to thirty minutes almost daily. I did this for years until I started studying in the field of health and fitness. Once I understood the benefits of getting physical exercise, I began trying new forms activity such as yoga, Chi Kung and taking classes at a gym. I even started hiking and running again! I have that doctor to thank for keeping me moving until I could develop a deeper passion for exercise. If you would like to start moving, walking is the best thing you can do for your health.

Studies show that physical activity *is inversely* related to the progressive buildup of plaque in the carotid artery leading to the heart. For lowering triglycerides, *a type of blood fat that raises heart attack risk*, accumulated ten minute segments of activity like walking and quick exercise are more effective than longer more continuous cardio workouts. Every bit of movement you do during the day burns calories and will help you get stronger.

Most people start exercising because it's "good" for them. But to stay motivated, you should know exactly why you want to start exercising. Compared with people who exercise regularly, *sedentary people are three times more likely to develop metabolic syndrome*—a combination of risk factors including high blood pressure (hypertension), elevated "bad" cholesterol, high blood sugar and obesity. Regular physical activity also has been found to reduce risk for cognitive decline. More reasons for motivation: People who regularly exercise live years longer and with a better quality of life than those who are sedentary. Aim to exercise briskly at an intensity that makes you perspire and breathe a little heavily while still being able to carry on a conversation.

Walking is man's best medicine. ~ Hippocrates

Walking is a convenient, affordable and enjoyable way to stay fit. Get a good fitting pair of walking or cross training shoes, warm up and you are ready to go. Here is why walking is the # 1 participation sport in the world:

- ♥ Improves muscle tone
- ♥ Eases back pain
- ♥ Lowers blood pressure
- ♥ Burns lots of calories and is the easiest way to lose weight
- ♥ Reduces risk of cancer, heart disease, stroke and diabetes

- ♥ Slows the progression of Alzheimer's and may prevent osteoarthritis
- ♥ Enhances energy, stamina and increases your aerobic capacity
- ♥ Lessens anxiety, tension and depression
- ♥ Easy on your joints
- ♥ Walkers live longer and enjoy physical and mental health benefits
- ♥ It is a great way to connect with friends and loved ones.
- ♥ Can be done when you travel, anywhere, anytime
- ♥ Help with sleep disorders
- ♥ Decreases your resting heart rate which means your heart has to work less and will last longer

How to Get Started:

- ♥ Make a game out of counting your daily steps. Buy pedometer, a wireless activity tracker or phone app such as "Map My Walk" to count your steps.
- ♥ Buy a new pair of athletic shoes that fit properly. There should be a thumb's width of space between your longest toe and the end of your shoe. The heel should not slip when you walk. Get help from a sales person. Make sure the shoes give you the support you need!
- ♥ Posture is crucial. *Keep your head up, spine straight and roll your shoulders back.*
- ♥ Remember to breathe regularly, taking deep breaths.
- ♥ Add steps to your daily routine by walking to the end of your driveway or road, doing errands on foot and going for three-ten minute walks per day.
- ♥ Take the stairs instead of the elevator. Park further away to get more steps in.
- ♥ Walk with friends or start a walking club. Try a walking meeting instead of sitting the whole time.
- ♥ Keep a journal or chart your progress.
- ♥ Remember to incorporate warm ups and then stretching to cool down.
- ♥ Drink enough water before, during, and after exercise.

Work up to a goal slowly. Start with ten minutes of walking per day until you reach thirty minutes per day. It doesn't matter how long it takes. Just beginning will build your self-esteem and give your more confidence.

Slow and Steady Wins the Race

A Pedometer or Tracking Device is Your Best Walking Buddy to Help You Lose Weight and Keep It Off

- **The 10,000 Step-A-Day Program** is a great program to get you started on your lifetime walking habit. This is a *goal to work up to for lasting health.*
- **To start**, most people find they walk 2,000 to 4,000 steps in a normal day- *but note—5,000 steps or less is considered sedentary living and harmful to your health.*
- **Health guidelines:** 30 minutes per day of brisk walking.
- **Fitness guidelines**: 60 minutes per day to manage body weight.
- **Weight loss guidelines**: 60 - 90 minutes per day of moderate intensity activity.

To convert steps to miles, here is a general guide, depending on your stride:

1. 10,000 steps = 5 miles
2. 5,000 steps = 2.5 miles
3. 2,500 steps = 1.25 miles
4. 1,250 steps = .625 (*Less than a mile*)

Inspire yourself to walk:
➢ If you walk 10,000 steps in a day you have walked 5 miles!
➢ If you walk 70,000 steps in a week you have walked 35 miles!

What a great goal! If you have a desk job, you may take less than 1,000 -5,000 steps per day. *This is considered sedentary living.* A walking program is essential for your well-being. You can fit in walks throughout your day by taking the stairs, walking a document to another department and walking at lunch. Breaking up walking throughout the day is more beneficial than you think!

♥ **Health Coach Wisdom:** "Walking 2 hours per week cuts your risk of dying early from cardiovascular disease by 53%," according to Harvard Medical School.

Tips for Walking Throughout Your Day

- ♥ Walk during your breaks.
- ♥ Take a walk at lunchtime.
- ♥ Take your shoes and stop to walk before you get home from work.
- ♥ Take the stairs instead of the elevator or escalator.
- ♥ Get off the bus or out of the taxi a few blocks before your destination.
- ♥ Take a walking vacation! Take a backpack and sightsee on foot!

Warm Up Before You Exercise to Prevent Injury

Warming up is one of the most important things you can do to prevent injury. A warm up is a slow rhythmic exercise of larger muscle groups performed before an activity that provides the body with a period of adjustment between rest and performance of that activity. Imitating an exercise activity for a period of 5 to 15 minutes before high intensity exercise improves overall performance. This technique gradually warms tissues, increasing blood flow and nutrients to active muscles, and prepares soft tissues for the flexibility needed for the activity. *You've probably heard this before, and if you are like most people, you ignore this advice because you are in a hurry and want to get going.* **Here are more reasons we need to warm up before exercising:**

- ♥ Increases your metabolism
- ♥ Increases muscle elasticity and **prevents injury**
- ♥ Increases flexibility of tendons and ligaments
- ♥ Limits lactic acid build up which causes soreness
- ♥ Increases speed
- ♥ Reduces risk of abnormal electrocardiogram
- ♥ Lubricates joints

Benefits of Strength Training

Strength training is the process of exercising with progressively heavier resistance for the purpose of strengthening the musculoskeletal system with these benefits:

- ♥ Four out of five Americans experience low back pain discomfort caused by being out of shape, having poor posture and using only certain muscles. Note that 80% of low back problems can be prevented by strengthening the lower back muscles.
- ♥ Enhances overall body composition and physical appearance

- Decreases resting blood pressure, increases metabolism and protects against a variety of degenerative problems
- Increases muscle size and strength–*making you stronger*
- Increases tendon and ligament strength–*helps prevent injuries*
- Increases bone strength–*helps prevent osteoporosis*

These changes have a profound influence on our physical capacity, physical appearance, metabolic function and injury risk. There are many ways to build strength. You can build strength by using your own body weight to do exercises such as push-ups, crunches, squats and lunges or you can lift weights or use resistance machines. *There are resources at the end of this chapter for ways to build muscle strength.*

Strong physical capacity allows us to perform work or exercise with less risk of injury and greater ease. Strength training increases the size and strength of our muscle fibers, resulting in a greater physical capacity to perform work. Stronger muscles enable us to lift a heavier weight once, which means muscle strength, while lifting a weight more than once means muscle endurance.

Strength Training Improves Physical Appearance

Our muscles have a lot to do with our overall physique. Strength training plays a major role in toning and shaping your body. When you lose fat and gain muscle, you will have a firmer and fit appearance. Unless we perform regular strength exercise, we lose more than one-half pound of muscle every year after the age of twenty-five. Without strength training, our muscles decrease in size and strength (atrophy). It is essential for preventing the muscle loss that accompanies the aging process. *To stay strong, we must engage in strength training exercises.*

Strengthening Our Muscles Boosts Our Metabolism

Muscle is very active tissue and burns calories even when we sleep! Skeletal muscles are responsible for more than 25% of calorie use. An increase in muscle tissue causes a corresponding increase in metabolic rate. Likewise, a decrease in muscle tissue causes a corresponding decrease in metabolic rate. In other words, *the more fit you are the more calories you burn, even long after your exercise session.*

Reduce your Risk of Injury and Pain

Our muscles serve as shock absorbers and balancing agents. Balanced muscle development reduces the risk of overuse injuries that result when one muscle group is much stronger than its opposing muscle group. Jogging, places more stress on the back leg muscles than the front leg muscles, creating a muscle imbalance that may cause knee injuries. A strength-training program that includes all the major muscle groups is an effective means of reducing the risk of injury and many degenerative diseases. Low back problems are often preventable by strengthening the lower back muscles. Building strength in all muscle groups helps prevent and relieve pain in all areas of the body.

Strength training has also been shown to:

- Increase mineral bone density–*making your bones stronger*
- Improve glucose metabolism–*helps you burn off the food you eat*
- Reduce gastrointestinal transit time–*aids digestion*
- Lower resting blood pressure–*good for your heart*
- Improve blood lipid levels–*a natural way to improve your blood tests*
- Ease arthritic pain–*lessen pain*

Why is Flexibility an Essential Part of Physical Fitness?

Flexibility training provides muscular relaxation, improves range of motion within joints, improves balance, speed, sports performance and reduces injury. Injuries occur as a result of tight or stiff muscles. Flexibility is the range of motion within a joint. A joint itself does not move; the body segments that come together within a joint move within the limitations of the joint. Within each joint and for each activity, there is an optimum ROM (Range of Motion) essential to peak performance. A number of factors can limit joint mobility: genetic inheritance; the joint structure itself, connective tissue elasticity within muscles, tendons or skin surrounding a joint strength of the opposing muscle group, and muscular coordination.

The Benefits of Flexibility

- Increased physical performance— *A flexible joint requires less energy to move through range of motion*
- Decreased risk of injury and pain
- Increased blood supply and nutrients to joint structures contributes to improved circulation greater elasticity of tissues
- Improved healthy synovial fluid also allows greater freedom of movement and may decelerate joint degenerative processes. *In other words, the synovial fluid in joint cavities helps alleviate pain from stiffness and arthritis.*
- Increased coordination

♥ Improved muscular balance and posture—*Flexibility helps realign soft tissue that may have adapted poor postural habits.* Stretching reduces the effort it takes to achieve and maintain good posture in activities and daily living.

♥ Decreased risk of low back pain

♥ Reduced muscular tension

♥ By relaxing both mind and body, flexibility training helps you feel better!

A Certified Personal Trainer will help assess your posture and structure a flexibility routine for you or you can also take a stretching class. Let the instructor know if you are a beginner, and don't compare yourself to others. Just be content where you are with each pose. It takes time to increase your flexibility.

The Mechanics of Stretching

♥ Start out slowly and take it easy

♥ Do not bounce

♥ Do not hold a stretch for too long when you are just starting

Static stretching involves a slow, gradual and controlled stretch through a full range of motion. To stretch, hold the pose until a gentle pull is felt, without pain for fifteen to thirty seconds. Most experts recommend a gentle stretch before and after intense activity. In preparation for activity, pre-stretch is primarily aimed at decreasing tissue stiffness, focusing particularly on the muscles that will be used. We want to stretch more after exercise to elongate the muscles, rather than before exercise because with intense exercise, body temperature increases and tissues offer less resistance

Factors affecting flexibility include age, gender, joint structure, muscle tendon attachments, body temperature, and pregnancy. Aging decreases our flexibility. A fair amount of dehydration in and around soft tissues also occurs as we age. This lack of water in soft tissue diminishes lubrication and the flow of nutrients to the site. The more active we are as we age, the more flexible we will be. Regular stretching can enhance flexibility and reduce natural wear and tear.

♥ **Health Coach Wisdom:** Remember that stretching for permanent elongation is best *after* your workout, not before. Most stretches should be held for a minimum of fifteen to thirty seconds and repeated two to three times each. *Slow and steady...*

Master Athlete Secret: "Top of the line, fitness keeps me fit at my age, and plays a huge role in staying engaged. It keeps me 100% full-out living. I take care of this body first," said Diana Nyad, sixty-four year old long distance swimmer who swam 111 miles from Cuba to Florida in fifty-two hours. "I love having an elevated spirit and being engaged with the planet more than the experience of swimming itself." She explained to Idea Fitness Journal that this engagement she feels, while gliding through the vast sea for hours on end with only the stars for company, is her secret to perpetual motion.

Cool Down After Every Type of Exercise

When we exercise we are usually in a hurry and want to skip the cool down. Here are a few reasons why it is so important to keep moving slowly while cooling down:

- ♥ Prevents blood from pooling after exercise and a quick drop in blood pressure, reducing the likelihood of post exercise lightheadedness or fainting
- ♥ Reduces the post-exercise tendency for muscle spasm, cramping and soreness
- ♥ Reduces exercise hormones immediately after vigorous aerobic exercise which lowers the probability of post-exercise disturbances in cardiac rhythm

Body Composition

Body composition is the last component of physical fitness. A healthy weight represents a healthy body composition. Our weight consists of body fat, and fat-free weight such as muscles, bones, blood, organs etc. When deciding on a healthy weight, we need to have a realistic understanding of how our bodies work and remember that getting fit is a journey, not a destination. Once you become fit and reach your healthy weight, you will want to maintain the healthy habits you have adopted to continue enjoying your healthy body. When you create a healthy lifestyle that you can sustain for life, you support yourself instead of creating a lofty goal that you work hard to achieve but then fall back into old patterns once you've achieved your target.

It is vital to understand that muscle weighs more than fat. I have worked with many clients who begin to eat more healthy and nutritious foods and exercise, yet become discouraged because they are not seeing the number on the scale change. What often happens is that while they are losing fat, they are toning and building muscle. I repeat: *Muscle weighs more than fat.* So even though people see their waist getting smaller and clothes fitting more loosely they get very upset at the number on the scale.

A few key things to consider:

- It took you a long time to put on the weight and it will take time to take it off.
- Muscle weighs more than fat and it will take time for your weight to drop
- If you are exercising you are gaining benefits in body and mind in a large number of ways. Relax and your weight will slowly go down.
- Have patience. Creating your healthy lifestyle includes everything in your life as a whole picture including all activity, exercising, eating well and relaxing.

The safest way to lose weight is to drop one to two pounds per week by balancing the amount of food energy in with the energy expended by moving.

♥ **Health Coach Wisdom:** The key to staying on your healthy path is *consistency!* Each day, make a plan for eating well and how you will get some activity. When you follow through on a consistent basis you create healthy habits. You will begin to see and feel the rewards in your body and mind. Just when my clients want to give up, I encourage them to stay the course—and it always pays off. Consistent small efforts provide great rewards!

From Surviving to Thriving

Renee was carrying a heavy box to the back room at work when she slipped, falling onto another box. Sandwiched between the thirty pound box she was holding and the carton below, Renee had fallen at an angle, injuring her spine. She was in terrible pain, but jumped up in embarrassment. Her back hurt so badly that she felt sick to her stomach, but she did not want to leave work before finishing her duties. She worked the rest of the day in excruciating pain before going home. The next morning she woke, barely able to move. She tried to get up and fell to the floor. She was rushed to the hospital, but the delay in getting medical care hurt her chances for recovery.

The next two years were some of the most difficult of Renee's life. The mother of two small children, she had injured her spine so severely that doctors told her she might never walk normally again. Renee was in constant pain, spending most of her days in bed ridden with guilt about not being able to take care of her family or work; she became depressed. Several months later she had gained so much weight that it became even more painful to move around. Her life was becoming unbearable.

That was twenty years ago. Today, Renee works, hikes, kayaks and fishes with her family. I interviewed Renee on a kayaking trip where she was teaching a group of women how to kayak on a local lake. I had heard of Renee's story and was interested to learn what gave her the ability to keep going and change her life. I asked her what motivated her do what she needed to do to survive, and what gives her the power to be healthy. "I wanted to be a part of life. I didn't want to miss out on anything. It was a long road back. I was in pain for much of my physical therapy, and after when I had to get out and start moving on my own. I bought a kayak with pedals and drove myself down to the lake as often as I could. It was not easy, but I was not going to let them convince me that I had to stay in a wheel chair."

"Renee", I asked, "so many people want to change, but they don't. What was it that made the difference for you?" She told me with great conviction, "I believed I could do it. I wanted to change. I did not want to live in pain and I came to the realization that I had to stop making excuses and start doing little things, one at a time. Many people look for a magic pill. Real change starts with our mental state. I understand that my weight and my health depend on my attitude. I came to see that my feelings and thoughts are directly related to my emotions. When faced with a choice, I ask myself if this fear is real or not. My thoughts can make me fearful, anxious or angry or I can focus on being positive instead of giving into fear, which allows me to enjoy life and gives me the ability to do the things I need to do to stay healthy."

Renee is one of the most inspiring people I have ever met. She overcame a series of difficulties in childhood, only to have a devastating accident after finally making it though the worst days of her life. Those who know her admire the fact that she still struggles with pain from her injuries, but she never complains and doesn't let it stop her from getting out, participating in life and contributing to her beautiful family, friends and community. She gives back by painting pictures of fallen solders for their families, training guide dogs and advocating for disabled people. She is a role model for so many of us with her positive can-do attitude.

Exercise is the Fountain of Youth

Being in good physical condition prevents injury while performing simple daily tasks, it prevents back pain and it prevents illness by strengthening the immune system. I have heard horror stories from countless people who ended up in tragic situations because they were not strong and became injured. This can become a slippery slope of illness, surgeries, becoming addicted to pain killers or exposed to super bugs that are too powerful to overcome. Lives are ruined and people can die as a result. The best way to prevent these tragedies is by being fit. In Renee's story, a random accident caused her injuries; however, she overcame her circumstances by doing whatever she needed to do to heal. The lesson here is that she followed through with the critical steps of her physical therapy, rose to the occasion and persevered.

Being physically fit helps you stay functionally fit, or keeping your body moving in ways nature intended it to so that you may perform daily activities. In order to perform simple tasks such as lifting children or bags of groceries, you need to have *muscular strength*. To carry a box from one place to another, you *need muscular endurance*. To bend over and reach for something you need to be *flexible*. To keep your heart strong and blood pumping you need *cardio respiratory* endurance. In order to perform daily tasks in a healthy manner and to be physically fit, you need to maintain a healthy body weight. What's more, exercising helps you to feel like a kid again!

What Do You Love To Do?

Do you love to walk outside and enjoy nature? Do you like to swim, play golf, water ski, play basketball, garden or cycle? Getting energy from activities you enjoy is your ticket to being fit. No matter how busy you are or what is on your "to do" list, you deserve time for yourself. Being active is important, so why not make it fun?

♥ **Health Coach Wisdom:** Put on exercise clothes first thing in the morning or pack your gym bag to take with you. No matter how your day unfolds, this confirms that you are going to do some form of exercise. It can be ten minutes of exercise before you take your shower or a link to whatever activity you choose that day. This tip works!

Another benefit of being active and exercising is burning calories. Using up calories allows you to eat a little more, provided you know what your body needs. Here is some incentive to get busy burning some energy:

Try something new!

Contrary to what most of us have been taught, exercise does not have to mean working hard or going fast. In fact, some of the most effective forms of exercise are based on slow methodical movements, such as yoga, tai chi, chi kung, Pilates and weight lifting.

The Benefits of Yoga are Limitless

Regular practice of yoga can help you face the turmoil
of life with steadiness and stability.
~ B.K.S. Iyengar

My yoga teacher, Patricia Carpizo Kauffman, pictured here, is one of the most beautiful and gentle women I have ever met. At the same time, she is stronger than most men. What is her secret? She has been practicing and teaching yoga, meditation and transforming emotions for over 25 years. The benefits of practicing Yoga are amazing. Patricia says:

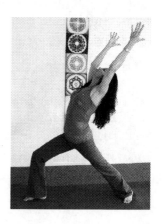

"Yoga is for everyone. Yoga helps to integrate the mental and the physical plane, and it offers a sense of inner and outer balance as well as alignment. Yoga activates all the muscles, bones, and organs of the body. It possesses the unique ability to calm the nerves, and has the holistic impact of relaxing the body and calming the mind. Yoga illuminates your life. Its light will spread to all aspects of your life. Regular practice will bring you to look at yourself and your goals in a new light. It will help remove the obstacles to good health and stable emotions. Yoga will help you achieve self-realization which is the ultimate goal of every person's life."

Yoga will help you remain flexible, help you to sleep better and encourages mindfulness. While many Westernized yoga classes focus on learning physical poses, look for an instructor who will also focus on breathing and meditation. Yoga increases your strength and balance while calming your nervous system. It has been proven to reduce heart disease, pain and anxiety and helps improve your posture.

What are Tai Chi & Chi Kung?

Tai Chi has a rich history. Experts believe it goes back well over 1,500 years. It is a gentle form of exercise for people of all ages as these movements help you gain strength, balance and flexibility. As a low-impact exercise, Tai Chi is great for people with joint problems because it can help strengthen connective tissue and improve circulation. Additionally, it improves balance and posture by emphasizing correct form. Tai Chi reduces tension and stress while improving body awareness. Chi Kung exercises are slow, fluid movements taught by the instructor that do not require memorizing a routine, yet help you to relax and focus.

> Your Dan Tien (abdomen) is the center of your body. It is what keeps you in balance. Bring the energy down from the sky and up from the earth to balance your health in harmony.
> ~Mariscela Alvarez, Tai Chi & Chi Kung Instructor

Sometimes called "meditation in motion," a Tai Chi workout is a series of soft, flowing movements choreographed into a slow routine. Each specific movement corresponds with either the inhalation or exhalation of a deep, gentle breath. This coordination of movement and breath is believed to free the flow of "chi" a life-force energy that when blocked, purportedly can cause stress and illness. By improving the mind-body connection, Tai Chi brings the yin and yang of a person back into natural harmony, exercising emotions just as it does the muscles.

Mariscela's advice for building a healthy lifestyle:

Know that you have the choice to create something different because your true nature is divine and the power is within you. Deep within, everyone holds a state of optimum health and inner-peace where all is well. Exercising your mind and body with Chi Kung and Tai Chi can help restore your health and well-being.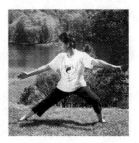

A Simple Guide to Beginning an Exercise Program

Check with your doctor before beginning any exercise program. Once you have been cleared, a simple way is to begin walking. As you feel comfortable, increase your distance, walk at a more brisk pace or increase the time of your walk.

Cross training or doing different types of exercise will help you to balance the muscle groups you are using. Walking is effective and by adding some resistance exercise by using your own body weight or lifting lift weights you begin to strengthen more muscle groups. Begin to do some light stretching after your exercise sessions to gain flexibility.

Setting Up Your Own Strength Training Program

Strength training is not advised for people with advanced heart disease, but healthy adults should do body weight exercises.

- Start with light 2, 3, 5 or 8 pounds weights. If you want to increase strength, do up to 12 repetitions. For muscular endurance, do more than 12 reps.
- For both goals, work up to three sets of 12 reps for each exercise. The American College of Sports Medicine recommends as a minimum: a) one set of 8 to 12 reps and, b) 8 to 12 exercises involving the major muscle groups of the body. Do these exercises twice per week. It can take as little as 10 minutes.
- Warm up by marching in place and doing some arm circles for about 5 minutes.
- Remember to breathe in and out while counting your reps and never hold your breath. (Inhale during the eccentric phase (bring the weight down) and exhale during the concentric phase (lifting or pushing the weight up-exertion).

Boost your strength by beginning an exercise routine. You can do this at home without any equipment. Strength exercises help flatten your belly and develop strength and definition in the hips and thighs. Be sure to find exercises that involve all major muscle groups: chest, shoulders, back, legs, arms, hips and trunk. **Here are a few examples of exercises to get you started.** For the first week, perform only one set of each exercise, resting at least thirty seconds before doing the next exercise. Try to do these exercises twice per week and once on the weekend for optimal results:

Glute Bridge: *Complete one set of 12 for at least one to two weeks. Increase over your time for a few weeks of training to reach your end goal of four sets of 12.*

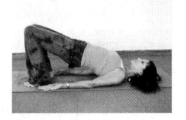

Lie on a mat on your back with your palms flat on the floor, your feet shoulder-width apart and your knees bent. Exhale as you press through your feet to lift your buttocks 3 to 6 inches off the floor. Push your pelvis up and hold for a few seconds, then slowly return to starting position.

Pushup: *If you have upper body strength, do a test to see how many PUSH UPS you can do to begin. Or start with the modified push up. Your goal should be to work up to 12 repetitions. After several weeks your goal could be to work up to four sets of 12 reps.*

Start with your arms extended but your elbows slightly bent. Your hands should be slightly wider apart than shoulder width; your fingers pointing forward, toes should be pointing down. Keep your head looking forward and slowly bend your elbows as you lower your chest to the floor. Keep your back straight and abdominal muscles tight. Stop when your elbows are even with your shoulders. Exhale and slowly raise yourself back to the starting position.

Modified or Knee push-ups: *Until you become comfortable, aim for 12 knee pushups. Build slowly over a few weeks until you reach a goal of four sets of 12 reps.*

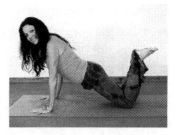

    Kneel on a mat on all fours with your knees hip-width apart, your hands slightly wider than shoulder-width apart, and your fingers pointing forward. Bring your pelvis forward so your body is in a straight line from your knees to your head. Inhale and lower your chest toward the floor until your elbows are even with your shoulders, keeping your abdominals tight. Exhale and push back to your starting position, keeping your elbows slightly bent, not locked.

Squat: *Complete one set of 12 repetitions. As you progress, add another set until after a few weeks you are comfortable with four sets of 12.*

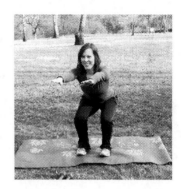

    Stand with your feet slightly wider than shoulder-width apart and your arms at your sides. Keep your back straight and abdominals tight then slowly squat down to about ninety degrees, exhaling as you go. Push your buttocks out as if you were going to sit in a chair. Make sure you don't let your knees extend forward past your toes to prevent injury to your knees. Inhale as you return to the starting position.

Front or Forearm Plank: *Hold for 5-20 seconds. Over time work up to 30-60 seconds. Do 2-3 sets.*

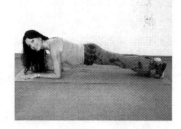

    Lay face down on the floor. Begin in the plank position with your forearms and toes on the floor. Keep your torso straight and your body in a straight line from ears to toes with no sagging or bending. Your head is relaxed and you should be looking at the floor in front of you.

Abdominal Crunch: *Do one set of 12. As you progress work toward four sets of 12.*

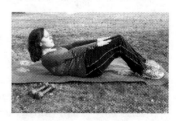

    Lie on your back with your knees bent and your feet flat on the floor. Place your hands across your chest or at your side. Without using your neck to raise you up, use your abdominal muscles, exhale and slowly curl your upper body off the ground until your shoulder blades are lifted up. Exhale as you slowly lower yourself to the starting position.

Reverse Lunge: *Do one set of 12 twice weekly, Slowly working up to four sets of 12.*

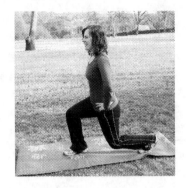

This low-intensity exercise, like the forward lunge, strengthens your quads, hamstrings, glutes, and calves. It's a great alternative to the forward lunge for those who are worried about knee injury, as it does not allow your knees to extend beyond your toes. *However, you should still be careful when performing this exercising, especially if you have a history of poor knees.* **Take a big step backwards with your left foot.**

Reverse Lunge continued: You should now be standing with your feet apart. **Lower your hips to the floor until your front (right) knee forms a 90-degree angle. Push yourself up.** Most of the strength should come from your front (right) foot. Return your back (left) foot to the starting position.

Chest Press w/Weights: *Do one set of 12 reps. Work up to four sets.*

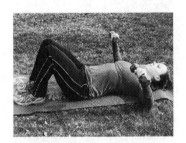

Lie on your back on a mat with your knees bent and your feet flat on the floor. Holding a weight in each hand, bring your elbows in line with your shoulders, making a right angle between your upper arm and your side. Exhale as you slowly extend your arms and press the weights up. Keep your elbows slightly bent. Inhale as you return to the starting point.

Tricep Overhead: *Using weights, perform one set of 12. Work up to four sets.*

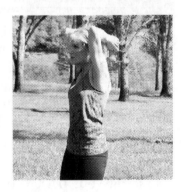

Stand with feet hip width apart, knees slightly bent. Grasp your weight with both hands and raise your arms over your head keeping your elbows slightly bent. Inhale as you slowly bend your elbows and lower the weight behind your head. Keep your elbows close to your head. When your forearms are parallel to the ground, exhale as you raise the weight to start position.

Cool-down

Stretches are designed to lengthen the muscles and relieve pain. Here are two examples, and you can find more resources at the end of this chapter. Hold each stretch for 20 seconds after you have done your workout.

Cat Camel

Get down on your hands and knees. Relax your head, and allow it to droop. Round your back up toward the ceiling until you feel a stretch in your upper, middle, and lower back. Hold stretch about 15 seconds. Return to the starting position with a flat back while you are on all fours. Let your back sway by pressing your stomach toward the floor and pushing your shoulder blades together. Hold for 15 seconds. Repeat 4 times.

Twist

Sit in a chair or on the floor facing forward. Take your right arm and place Your elbow or hand to the outside of your left knee. Look behind you over your left shoulder until you feel a twist in your spine. Hold for 15 seconds. Repeat other side.

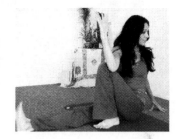

Following is an example of a simple one month plan:

Monday	Cardio: Brisk Walk 10 minutes
Tuesday	Strength Using Body and Weights: 10 minutes
Wednesday	Cardio: Brisk Walk: 10 minutes
Thursday	Strength Training: Exercises 10 minutes
Friday	Cardio: Brisk Walk 10 minutes
Saturday	Exercise Class: Yoga, Stretching or Chi Kung 30-60 minutes
Sunday	Sport: Golf, Bicycle, Tennis, Swimming 30-60 minutes

Week One: follow specified times.
Week Two: add five minutes to your cardio and increase your sets of exercises.
Week Three: increase to 15 minutes of walking or cardio. Add exercise sets.
Week Four: increase walking to 20-30 minutes. Remember, you can break the walking up into 10 minute sessions. Increase weights and sets of exercises.

♥ **Health Coach Wisdom:** More than 40% of Americans will experience a serious balance disorder, according to the National Institute of Health. Bad balance causes falls, which are a leading cause of death among seniors. **The ideal way to develop better balance is to strengthen muscles throughout your body. You can stay strong if you exercise your muscles!**

Understanding Your Exercise Heart Rate

There are numerous methods for monitoring exercise intensity. It is important for you to be familiar with your heart rate while exercising so you can know your limits. The easiest way to measure exercise intensity is by a method known as the **Rate of Perceived Exertion (RPE).** In this method, you estimate your exercise exertion by assigning it a number. In recent years a revised scale has made it easier to use with a rating of 0 to 10.

Rating	Explanation
0	Nothing at all
.5	Very, very weak
1	Very weak
2	Weak
3	Moderate
4	Somewhat strong
5	Strong
6	
7	Very strong
8	
9	
10	Very, Very Strong
	Maximal Heart Rate

To obtain your **Resting Heart Rate,** take it first thing in the morning before rising. Count the number of beats of your heart for 30 seconds and multiply by 2 to get your resting heart rate. Resting heart rate in adults is usually 60 to 100 beats per minute and is regular in rhythm. *Well-trained endurance athletes have developed an efficient cardiovascular system and often have resting heart rates in the low 40s. If an untrained person's resting heart rate is greater than 100 or less than 60, or if the heart rate is irregular, they should get checked by their doctor.*

♥ **Health Coach Wisdom:** Listening to music is a great way to get moving faster, to raise your heart rate. It really helps to inspire you, lift your mood, and will give you extra energy for a better workout!

To determine your Maximal Heart Rate use this mathematical calculation:

220–(minus) your age = max heart rate

Note: You should use caution when figuring your Max heart rate with the 220-your age formula as it has a variability of 10-12 beats per minute depending on several factors.

Percentage of Maximal Heart Rate: This method of monitoring intensity of exercise calculates the exercise heart rate as a percentage of maximal heart rate. You can use the following formula:

Training Heart Rate = maximal heart rate x desired percent of max heart rate, such as, 55 or 65% to 90%.

For example, if you are 50 years old: 220-50= 170. (Your max heart rate)

170 X 65% = 110.5

Here is an easy way to determine your heart rate when exercising:

1. Get a stopwatch or watch with a second hand, then find your pulse. You can locate your pulse either in your radial artery on your wrist or at your carotid artery in your neck. Choose the spot that works best for you.
2. To measuring your heart rate, you must use the correct fingers to do the measuring. Your thumb has a light pulse and can create confusion when you are counting your beats. It's best to use your index finger and middle finger together.
3. After you find the beat, you need to count how many beats occur within 60 seconds. The shortcut to this method is to count the number of beats in 10 seconds, and then to multiply that number by 6. This method gives you a 60-second count.
4. For example, after walking up hill, stop and find your pulse. Look at your second hand and count the number of beats in 10 seconds—if you counted 18 then multiply that number by 6 and you will get 108.

Physical Activity Intensity

To figure your *target heart rate*:

Figure your max heart rate (220 - your age) =_____.

Multiply your max heart rate: _____ x .5 (or 50%) =_____.

Multiply your max heart rate: _____ x .7 (or 70%) =_____.

These two numbers are your training zone. Do not exercise or work out at your maximum heart rate! You should change it up and move within your zone. *Most importantly, exercise at a pace in which you feel comfortable.*

To develop a strong cardiovascular system, aim to reach 50% to 85% of your maximum heart rate for at least 30 minutes, five days a week. If you don't do any type of exercise at all, you will need to work up to this slowly.

♥ **Health Coach Wisdom:** Moving around during the day is one of the best things you can do for your health. To prevent or control type 2 Diabetes and heart disease, *move at least 5 minutes out of every 55 that you sit.* Physical activity helps your insulin do its job and absorbs glucose from the bloodstream. ***Three five minute walks can equal a dose of medication for people with type 2 diabetes!*** *(Do not skip medication. This is from a recent study to illustrate the power of exercise.)*

Help for Those Stuck in the Office

People who work in an office environment have it tough, especially if they don't have the freedom to get up and move around. This type of sedentary lifestyle is killing Americans. Create the mindset that you will get up from your chair at every opportunity. You can stand while talking on the telephone, walk to drop off paperwork at someone's office instead of e-mailing. Take the stairs. During your workday, get outside to get some fresh air and sunshine which produces vitamin D. On breaks, and even at your desk, follow these simple exercises to help prevent and relieve pain:

- **Breathe** in through the nose and out through the mouth.
- **Breathe deeply:** Be in the present moment.
- **Posture:** Sit up straight, yet relaxed in shoulders, back, knees
- **Neck**: look left then right, breathing 6 times
- **Neck**: gently look up, then down, slowly, breathing 6 times
- **Head tilt**: ear to shoulder 6 times
- **Roll finger tips on back of neck** to remove knots and tension
- **Shoulder rolls**: 6 back, 6 forward
- **Arm and shoulder flexibility test:** Lift right arm up overhead palm face back then touch your back. With your left hand reach around and touch your right fingers. Repeat on other side.

- **Side twists:** sitting forward, twist to the right facing behind you putting your right hand on the back of the chair. Breathe deeply and hold. Repeat on other side.
- **Point and flex toes**, 6 each
- **Pick up each knee:** hug into chest for 15 seconds
- **Pain reliever**: Clasp hands behind you then touch palms
- **Side stretches:** Lift right arm overhead and lean to the left. Repeat other side.
- ***Go to my website for more desk exercises!*** *www.lynellross.com*

♥ **Health Coach Wisdom:** *The biggest mistake we make is to "wait" to become active or eat healthy.* Don't wait until next week or after a holiday, do something today! Do something every day to become fit.

Action Steps

What vision do you have for your fitness? Think about what picture you envision and why it is important to you. What will you look and feel like? Why is it important to you? Write your vision in your journal or here: _____

_____

_____

_____.

What steps can you take to achieve your fitness goals? Remember to work on one thing at a time and keep the steps small and realistic.

Examples for beginners:

- *I will walk three times this week for ten to fifteen minutes on Saturday, Monday and Wednesday.*
- *I will do strength exercises for ten minutes on Tuesday and Thursday and attend a yoga class on Friday.*
- *I will buy a treadmill or elliptical for home and use it three times a week for fifteen minutes on Monday, Wednesday and Friday.*
- *I will join a nearby gym or fitness center this month to learn more about fitness.*

Pick one small fitness goal for the week and write it here:

_____.

Write down one healthy fitness habit to develop this month:

_____.

- *It takes 28 days to form a new habit, so concentrate on this action daily.*

Write down an affirmation around fitness that means something to you:

_____.

Here is my favorite exercise affirmation:

Every day that I exercise is a great day!

♥ **Health Coach Wisdom:** *Exercise with the seasons!* Beware of the pitfall of engaging in an exercise you are really happy with, only to have the weather change with the seasons. It is a pleasure to go out for a walk in the spring, but when summer temperatures soar, or winter storms hit, it is difficult to walk outside and you lose momentum. Be prepared to shift into a new exercise routine with a plan for every season. Buy a treadmill for home, join a gym or use exercise DVDs to stay on track during extreme hot or cold temperatures. Plan ahead.

Use "My Fitness Calendar" at the end of this chapter to keep track of your minutes of activity. Log your minutes of actual exercise *and* minutes spent on extra things such as mowing the lawn, cleaning house, working in the garden and walking while shopping. This is the best way to actually see many minutes you are moving. *If you go several days without walking or exercising it will become obvious to you.*

Every choice starts a behavior that over time becomes a habit.
~ Darren Hardy

Fitness resources for you:

www.acefitness.org: The American Council on Exercise provides free fitness instruction, healthy recipes and cutting edge health information.

www.acsm.org: The American College of Sports Medicine for fitness information.

www.JorgeCruise.com: Jorge Cruise "8 Minutes in the Morning Kit" comes complete with exercise cards picturing exercises with easy instructions, a CD and booklet.

www.fitdeck.com: Exercise playing cards with hundreds of exercises broken down by exercise type illustrated with easy to follow instructions. Makes exercising fun!

www.walkathome.com: Leslie Sansone is a nationally recognized fitness expert who created the Walk at Home Program, a simple and fun way to get moving anytime!

wwwlynellross.com: For more fitness tips and exercise tips, exercise programs, healthy recipes and stress management ideas.

www.fyspirit.com: Mariscela Alvarez' Tai Chi and Chi Kung exercise DVDs, information on guided meditations and hypnotherapy.

My Fitness Calendar for: _____

Each day write down the minutes & type of exercise or steps you take to keep you motivated and active.

Sunday	Monday	Tuesday	Wednesday	Thursday	Friday	Saturday

I am strong, fit and healthy so that I can do things I enjoy

My exercise goal for this month is: _____

My nutrition goal for this month is: _____

My plan to reduce stress is: _____

Chapter 4

Be Socially Connected in a Healthy Way

The quality of your life is the quality of your relationships.
~Tony Robbins

Why do some people thrive while most people merely survive? Being well and thriving does not happen by chance. Each of the eight steps to vibrant health in the model for wellness I found while creating this book are tied to one another. Being connected to other human beings in a healthy way is a key link in the chain of wellness that brings joy, satisfaction and wholeness.

When people are angry, stressed or having conflicts in relationships, they are the least likely to focus on their health. In turn, this makes them feel bad, rendering them unable to be their best around others. Do unhealthy relationships cause stress or does stress create poor relationships? Both can be true, and one thing is certain: If you are experiencing trouble in your closest relationships, it will take a toll on your health. If you have strong and healthy relationships you are more likely to thrive.

Close relationships with your friends, family and community make you feel safe, and is linked to a longer life according to a Brigham Young University analysis including more than 300,000 people. Decades of research show that when people are in stable and healthy marriages, they live longer. Relying on a best friend or having a circle of friends does wonders for your health, including improved heart health, less chance of depression and increased ability to heal. "People who have a strong social network have 50% less heart disease than those who are lonely," according to Dr. Lissa Rankin.

Before we can cultivate solid relationships with others, we need to develop a good relationship with ourselves. When you learn to love yourself, and be your own best friend, you will have more love to give away. But just how is that possible?

♥ **Health Coach Wisdom:** When you put your health first, you are more prepared to deal with the stressors in your life and change your own self-defeating behaviors. When you are thriving and happy, you are not likely to create or bring drama into your life, helping you to heal your relationships.

Self-Esteem – Finding our Best Self

What is Self-Esteem? Self-Esteem means truly loving and valuing yourself. This is not arrogant. In fact, those who boast the loudest are often most desperately lacking in true-self esteem. Good self esteem means that you:

- ♥ Accept yourself as you are
- ♥ Give yourself credit for the things you do
- ♥ Take time to recognize your accomplishments
- ♥ View problems and challenges as opportunities
- ♥ Learn from failures and see them as chances to grow
- ♥ Have a healthy self image *no matter what your title or economic status*
- ♥ Value what you think over what other people think

How do you begin to build your self-esteem? One answer is to consciously be kind, compassionate and forgiving with yourself. What we think about ourselves becomes what we believe. It's not what others say about us, it is what we say about ourselves that matters. If you think you are unworthy, you'll never feel good about yourself.

If you love yourself, others will find you loveable and you will be able to love them back. Your self-concept accepts whatever you choose to believe and selects experiences to prove that belief. If you don't believe you deserve to be happy, then you won't be happy. Your subconscious mind takes your beliefs and creates habits built on them.

Social Connections Create Authentic Happiness

When my second son was born, I was afraid that I would not be a good boy's mom. However, I soon came to realize that having sons was a gift. I learned how to become a good mother to my sons, enjoying all the new adventures I had not known as a child, including soccer, baseball, basketball, hiking, camping and fishing. I appreciated how simple it was to make boys happy. Good food and a variety of activities was all it took to bring beaming smiles. I especially loved the way that boys didn't sweat the small stuff; there was no drama in our home, only lots of laughter.

As my sons grew, I began to bond with a group of women who were also boys' moms. Perhaps it was because we identified with the endless loads of dirty laundry and uniforms to wash. Maybe it was helping each other with new recipes to feed the voracious appetites of teams of boys roaming through the house. Mostly it was to fill the need for female companionship that created our lasting friendships. By the time my last son was about to graduate from high school, this small group of women had become as close as any friends could be. I worried about us because our sons were all going away at the same time, leaving us with empty nests. Being a planner, I called upon my Life Coach to help us through this difficult time. After the boys were all settled at college, we had our first meeting. We were nervous to talk about our feelings, but willing to at least show up for each other.

Our Life Coach began by teaching us listening skills, boundary setting and being able to open up and speak the truth about our feelings. It was a little uncomfortable at first, but the act of revealing how we really felt, opening up and being vulnerable to one another helped us to create a bond of trust. We learned what a great feeling it is to have friends to call upon when you need them and knowing you will be there for each other without judgment. It's even better to be there to help your friends when they need support. We have no jealousy in our group, no one gossips about the other and we are there for each other no matter what happens. I do not think that our friendships would have been strengthened after the kids left if we had not taken the step to bring in a qualified coach to help us learn how to be better friends, better listeners and better human beings who aim to live without judging. None of us feels lonely, even when we miss our kids, because we always have someone there who understands.

I have watched these types of friendships throughout my life. One of the qualities I admired most about my mother-in-law, Katherine, was her love of her friends. During her lifetime she kept in contact with friends from kindergarten to college. She kept weekly or monthly dates with these groups after she retired from teaching. With one group she played bridge weekly, one group met yearly at a friend's cabin, one met for tennis and lunch. She was always traveling with friends for great fun and new adventures.

When she was in her late seventies, she was still very active until she became ill with shingles. Her activity level declined and she lost her muscle mass, becoming quite weak. My mother-in-law passed away after falling and breaking a hip. She had contracted the super bug MRSA in the hospital. This happened suddenly, and we had no time to contact all her friends. I was *the first one back at her house and saw the light blinking on her answering machine.*

Wanting to spare my husband and his brothers the pain of listening to the messages, I sat down at her desk and began the task of listing the names and numbers of the callers. Listening to each message became more and more gut wrenching, with each friend crying out, "What has happened? Where are you? I heard you were in the hospital. Are you all right? We have our trip coming up next month and we can't plan this without you. You always plan everything. We don't know what to do without you." By the time I had finished listening to the last message, I could barely see though my tears. I sat at her desk for the longest time, sobbing until I had a headache. The love that her friends had for her was as strong as any sister.

A few years later when I attended memorial services for my cousin and for a close friend, both of whom had died from heart problems, I became acutely aware of the special bonds of friendship. Friend after friend spoke at each of these services about the great times they had together, reciting stories in detail about the everyday adventures that made up their lives. As I drove home from my dear cousin's memorial, I thought about his friends and how they knew him so well. I realized that close friends bring out the best in each other and how when we are with them we are our truest selves.

If you are a person that has close friends, or if you belong to clubs and organizations, then you already understand. If you stay to yourself or feel lonely, you might consider how you can expand your circle to include a few more friends, join a club, or volunteer where you can be around others and make new friends. Your heart will benefit from opening up to others.

When you have the choice to be right or be kind, pick kind.
~ Dr. Wayne Dyer

How Your Self Awareness Affects Your Relationships

We human beings are particularly good at pointing out the flaws of others. We label and judge others. However, when someone tries to tell us where to make changes, we can become indignant, angry and defensive, or even deny that the problem exists.

When we become self-aware we begin to build better relationships. We can start understanding our own behavior by keeping a journal, reading books, seeing a therapist or working with a coach. Each of us has positive strengths and negative traits which become a part of our story, yet we may hold beliefs about ourselves that are in our subconscious. We may not even be aware of these judgments. We may also find fault with ourselves without taking time to praise ourselves for our strengths. We may feel that we don't measure up and often feel shame and guilt.

Emotional Intelligence is first being aware of the motives and feelings of other people and yourself, and secondly knowing how to fit into different social situations. *Emotional Intelligence is the key to understanding others.* If you don't know how you feel or why you feel a certain way, you may not be able to communicate effectively or resolve disagreements. We are born happy, kind and loving, yet with the passage of time, we form personalities. When we believe that these personalities rule us, we may have trouble with other people. Have you ever said *"That's just the way I am?"* It is possible to change the way you think about yourself and it doesn't have to take a long time. You only need to be courageous enough to look at your actions in an objective way. If you want to be more kind, loving, forgiving, open, flexible, courageous or any other trait you desire, you can expand these strengths. You already possess all good traits; *you only need to believe it. We also possess the negative traits. When we are aware of them, they lose their power over us.* If your goal is to improve your relationships then it helps to be aware of various strengths and personality types in you and others. *Read this list and gently notice what comes up for you while being accepting of all traits.*

Positive Traits	Negative Traits or Thoughts
Kind	Unkind
Loving	Unloving/coldhearted
Honest	Untruthful
Forgiving	Unforgiving
Aware	Unconscious
Other Centered	Self-centered
Giving	Selfish
Compassionate/Social Intelligence	Unfeeling/Unaware of other's feelings
Brave/courageous	Cowardly/afraid
Smart/witty	Stupid/unthinking
Careful/prudent/cautious/responsible	Reckless/irresponsible
Wise/thoughtful/non-reactive	Unthoughtful/reactive
Appreciative /grateful	Ungrateful
Leader/doer	Blind follower /do nothing
Perseverance	Quitter

Positive Traits	Negative Traits or Thoughts
Curious/open	Closed off/closed minded/prejudiced
Fair /inclusive	Unfair /exclusive
Energetic	Lazy
Non Judgmental	Judgmental
Humble	Arrogant/Grandiose /superior
Self-disciplined	Lacking self regulation or discipline
Spiritual	Alone
Teamwork/sharing the load/work for good of group	Sense of Entitlement/ work only for yourself
Creativity	Dullness/lacking spark/closed off
Humorous /bring smiles to others/see light	Humorless/ bring pain to others /see dark

He who knows others is wise. He who knows himself is enlightened.
~ Lao-tzu

Alan Cohen, Life Coach, author and spiritual teacher in his book, *The Dragon Doesn't Live Here Anymore–Living Fully, Loving Freely,* helps us to understand our own positive and negative traits and how we relate to other people:

> There is nobody out there. All that we see are reflections, or mirror images of our own self. When we talk, we are only talking to our self. When we fight, we only fight our self. When we love, we are only giving love to self. There is only One Being in all the universe and It is Us.
>
> Most of the time, the trait against which we are reacting to in another is something within our self that we do not accept. If you make a list of the positive and negative traits of someone you don't like, you will probably find a striking number of similarities between them and yourself. This requires a great deal of honesty, but if you can do it with a high intention, you will grow tremendously from it.

This is why we feel so bad when we speak negatively about someone else, when we judge, when we fight or yell at someone. We are hurting ourselves as we hurt others. When we are annoyed at another's actions, we are really annoyed at ourselves because somewhere inside we have the same trait and have said or done the same type of thing. If you get very still and very honest with yourself you will recognize it.

A big lesson I have learned is that the things that bother me most about other people are things that I have denied about myself. I disliked those traits so much, that I was blind to the fact that I indeed possessed and showed them. When I spent the time to quietly assess each trait, I found an example of where I had been at times both on the positive side and on the negative side. This produced a huge shift that I felt deeply. Our ego does not want to admit when we are wrong or when we have done something we are not proud of. The irony here is that other people see it and we don't! Imagine that. We think we are hiding that dark side or we don't even know we are doing something annoying or hurtful, but other people can see it clearly. They either: 1) tell us about what we just did or said and how it hurt them, and we may not only deny it, or we get angry at them for pointing it out, or 2) they don't tell us, which is worse. They quietly become annoyed or angry with us and if we keep up the bad behavior, they may shut us out altogether. If enough of our friends cut us out of their lives or distance themselves from us, it is time to look at our own behaviors instead of blaming others. This thought motivates me to want to understand my own behavior and examine the things I say and do more carefully while being aware of the reasons for my emotions. Awareness is the key to being compassionate with ourselves and others.

♥ **Health Coach Wisdom:** I've read that you become like the five people you spend the most time with. Choose wisely. Are your friends living a healthy and happy lifestyle? Are you setting a good example?

When you start to increase your awareness you become more honest with yourself from a place of compassion. Blame and judgment against yourself will only serve to hurt you or keep you blinded to your negative traits. When you are compassionate with yourself, you will be open to the truth, handle change more easily and be more patient with yourself and others.

♥ **Health Coach Wisdom:** Try to find the balance between serving others while taking care of yourself. Self-care is not selfish, it is imperative. If you feel good, you will be able to help others. Find your balance by making a daily list of all the things you need to do for your health. After that add things to the list that supports someone else.

Then carry out your tasks with a light heart. *Go to my website for a free downloadable Daily Wellness Checklist. www.lynellross.com.*

Focus on the Positive

Now consider your strengths more carefully. What are your positive traits? All of us possess some these traits to the degree that we accept them: Kind, loving, a leader, hopeful, fair, honest, humble, spiritual, creative, humorous, courageous. When we focus on the positive we are more able to make changes. When you are aware of your own behavior you will have more control over how you react to others. Once you discover your limiting beliefs and self-defeating behaviors you will be free to live the life you want. You will treat others the way you would like to be treated.

In the book "*The Power of Kindness: the Unexpected Benefits of Leading a Compassionate Life*" Piero Ferrucci, explains the importance of social connection and a sense of belonging:

> The sense of belonging-that is, the feeling that we are part of a whole greater than ourselves, with which we are physically, mentally and spiritually involved-is a necessary factor to our well-being. When we feel isolated, we will seek some affiliation at all costs, even with groups that are violent, dangerous, and extremist. This is one of the reasons many adolescents are attracted by gangs.

> The love I invest in my relationships returns to me multiplies many times over.
> ~ Alan Cohen, author, speaker, Life Coach

There are many studies that conclude that as much as we have the need to be individuals, we also have the need to connect with others. Additionally, we are happier when we are inclusive and open with people from all areas of life. Rather than being closed off to your immediate circle, be open to meeting new people, extending a hand when needed and looking for the best in others. *You will find whatever you are looking for.*

Piero Ferrucci explains,

> We are made of our perceptions. What we see or presume to see day after day constitutes who we are and colors our entire life. If our view is tired and stale and if everything we see appears empty, we will end up empty shells ourselves. If we see people as interesting and special, our world becomes stimulating and open. We also become more relaxed.

When people are angry their blood pressure and heart rate increase. Yet, when we feel appreciation for one another, our heart rate slows, blood pressure decreases and a parasympathetic response is created which has shown to be very protective to the heart.

> The choice to follow love through to its completion is the choice to seek completion within ourselves. The point at which we shut down on others is the point at which we shut down on life. We heal as we heal others, and we heal others by extending our perceptions past their weaknesses. Until we have seen someone's darkness, we don't really know who that person is. Until we have forgiven someone's darkness, we don't really know what love is. Forgiving others is the only way to forgive ourselves, and forgiveness is our greatest need. ~Marianne Williamson

What are your barriers to being more socially connected?

- Do you have a problem with clutter? Are you isolated from having friends and family to your home?
- Do you consider yourself shy and find it hard to join a club or organization?
- Do you have a problem getting along with others at work or at home?

If you want to improve your relationships, there are no shortages of information and help. There are books and courses, or you may consider hiring a life coach or therapist who can help you to identify areas that are holding you back. In his book *Nonviolent Communication*, Marshal B. Rosenberg, PhD, teaches us how to transform our thinking and moralistic judgments to improve the quality of our relationships. He explains how to speak, think, and listen in ways that inspire compassion and understanding. *No matter what difficulties you are having, Rosenberg's work will help you heal your relationships.*

Consider supportive counseling services to help with anxiety, depression or difficult relationships. Taking one action step will help you from feeling stuck. A good therapist can help you by looking back at your life, bringing to light troubles that are keeping you trapped in habits that do not serve you.

> Any fool can criticize, condemn, and complain-and most fools do.
> ~ Dale Carnegie

Dealing with Anger and Conflict

We all face conflict in our lives. It is a normal part of life and natural in relationships, from friends and family to co-workers or classmates. It is how we deal with conflict that's important. Sometimes conflict happens because people believe they have different goals *when really they have the same goal.* We may just have different personalities or styles. That's why communication is the key to solving conflict.

When we are in a conflict with someone and are angry, we need to learn to deal with anger in a positive way. No matter what someone else does, learning how to manage angry feelings is our responsibility. When we are angry and defensive, we are not able to hear others or think clearly. When we learn to work out our differences, we can overcome difficulties and make our relationships stronger.

Alcohol and other drugs usually make conflict worse. Some people turn to alcohol or drugs to help them cope with their problems, or mask their feelings. Not only won't alcohol or drugs help you solve problems, they increase the risk of violence and addiction. At the very least, they impair your judgment and cause you to say things you regret. *If you live with someone with a drug or alcohol problem, seeking help for yourself will help to empower you. See the list of resources at the end of the chapter for help.* Improving your communication skills is the best thing you can do to prevent and resolve conflict.

When you are faced with a conflict, remember these strategies:

- **Manage your anger** and calm down by walking away or deep breathing.
- **Define the problem.** Determine what you are really upset about and what your end goal is.
- **Communicate well.** When you take the time to talk with the other person in a **calm respectful way**, you can work together to solve the problem.
- **Do not try to reason with a person who is under the influence of alcohol or drugs.** You are not talking with them; *you are talking to the drugs or alcohol.* Remain calm and seek help for yourself. Remove yourself from the situation.
- **See through to the person's spirit.** The person you are in conflict with will see themselves as you see them. If you see their goodness and ask them questions that will help them understand and communicate what they want, they will soften their position and you will be able to understand each other.

Deep Breathing Will Calm Your Mind and Body

Try this exercise to calm down when you feel yourself getting angry or anxious:

- ♥ Sit comfortably or lie on your back
- ♥ Breathe in slowly and deeply through your nose for a count of 5.
- ♥ Hold your breath for 3-5 seconds.

- ♥ Breathe out slowly through your mouth for a count of 5, *slowly release the air.*
- ♥ Repeat until you feel calm and relaxed.

Every yoga session ends with a relaxation pose called Shavasana, which is perhaps the most important part of yoga practice. *I began practicing this at home whenever I felt upset, and it helped me become aware of my heart rate, which immediately calmed me down. You can try this anytime*: Lying on your back, relax your arms and legs placed at about a 45 degree angle. Close your eyes breathe deeply. Relax your entire body with an awareness of each breath. Scan all parts of your body for muscular tension, then release as it is found. Relax your breath, your mind, and body for a few minutes. Shavasana allows the body a chance to reset itself. The physiological benefits of yoga and deep relaxation are numerous and include:

- ♥ Decreases heart rate, blood pressure and muscle tension
- ♥ Reduces general anxiety and the number and frequency of anxiety attacks
- ♥ Increases energy levels and general productivity
- ♥ Improves concentration, memory and increase in focus
- ♥ Decreases fatigue, and helps with deeper more sound sleep
- ♥ Improves self-confidence.

11 Keys to Better Relationships

Not having close friends or confidants is as detrimental to your health as smoking or carrying extra weight. ~ Kate Larson, Executive Coach

Be honest with yourself: Being honest means having integrity. Abraham Lincoln defined *character* as *"Doing the right thing when no one else is looking."* If you always try to do the right thing, then you will be proud of yourself helping you to make good choices. When being honest with others, *do so carefully.* Ask yourself if it will hurt or help. When you get to know and trust yourself, you will be sensitive to others while being honest which creates better relationships.

Practice good communication: Listen to what the other person is saying. When you refrain from judging, criticizing or interrupting and give the other person your full attention, they will be more likely to listen and understand you. How does it make you feel when you are talking to someone and they are looking everywhere but at you? Successful people always look others in the eye, helping them to feel valued.

Seek first to understand, then to be understood. ~ Stephen R. Covey.

Treat others with kindness: Before you speak, ask yourself, "How would I like to be treated in this situation?" Check your tone of voice. How are you speaking to those around you? If you are asked a question, answer it promptly and politely, showing respect for others. Don't criticize; nothing shuts down communication faster than criticism. No one wants to be criticized, yet we can be very quick to judge and tell others what they "should have done." *No one wants to hear that.*

Learn how to say no: Throughout your life, people will ask you to do things that you do not want to do. Part of maturing is knowing the difference between helping somebody when they need it and deciding whether you can help them without hurting yourself. Saying no can be difficult because we don't want to disappoint people. Stand up for yourself as you would others. If you need to say no, just say so without explaining yourself. If you must give an answer, tell the truth politely and keep it simple. When you say no, most people do not care why, and you are not obligated to tell them. It is better to be fair and honest without keeping others hanging.

Do not take things personally: This is hard to understand and even harder to practice, but usually other people are thinking about themselves. The comment or judgment they make about you comes from their opinion of themselves. *The message to you is to stop worrying about what others think.* What matters is what *you* think of *yourself.* Your communication with others will improve when you are not snapping at them for things they've said which "upset you." If there is some truth, consider how you can grow and do something about it.

Be grateful and show appreciation: Look around you and be grateful for all you have. When you take time to appreciate your health, your home, your family, your friends, pets, and your abilities—you will be a happier person. Even better, take the time *to tell others* when you appreciate them. Thank people who have done things for you. Give credit to others where credit is due. Always remember to say thank you and you will not only make someone's day, but they will appreciate you for it.

Take responsibility for your own actions: Learn from your own mistakes. If something goes wrong, instead of beating yourself up, learn from what happened. Do not blame others. Take responsibility for yourself. Apologize if you can and learn the lesson. Don't obsess about it or feel sorry for yourself. See it as a learning experience and be confident that you will do better next time. Making a mistake is an opportunity to learn. Your relationships will blossom when you stop blaming.

Realize that your mood affects others: You might be stressed, worried, tired, hungry, sad or angry, but if you take your bad mood out on others, it hurts everyone, including yourself. If you are upset or having a problem, tell those around you that you need some time by yourself, but do not lash out at them. Trust those you love to honor your wishes. Take time to be quiet and ask yourself what is really upsetting you and find solutions. Ask for help when you need it.

Think positively: No matter what the circumstances are, try to see the positive side and appreciate the lesson. Ask "What can I learn from this?" Learn to be flexible. If your plans have to change, consider how you can make things better. *You get what you think about.* If you believe you can do something, and work at it, you will know you have done your best. If you want a positive relationship, then be positive. Think good thoughts. Learn how to calm yourself down and go inside to find an inner peace. Trust yourself to handle any situation and you won't have to worry about trusting others to meet your expectations.

Build a social support group: There is nothing more rewarding than sharing life with people you love and respect. Surround yourself with your own "Dream Team", people you love, good friends, family, co-workers, mentors and professionals who you rely on for advice and understanding. *Then give back to them.*

Accept other people for who they are: The only person you have control over is you. Trying to change someone else is never appreciated. When you change, others around you may shift because they are inspired by you. Don't offer advice. Allow people to figure things out for themselves. Each of us is wise when we listen to our best self.

> It is not insult from another that causes your pain. It is the part of your mind that agrees with the insult. Agree only with the truth about you, and you are free.
> ~ Alan Cohen, Author

If you want to improve your relationship with someone, remember these tips:

- ♥ Listen well to what they are saying and feeling, be open
- ♥ Treat them with respect
- ♥ Be kind, thoughtful, loving, non-judgmental and non-attached
- ♥ Spend time together doing activities they like
- ♥ Support their goals, hopes and dreams without giving advice
- ♥ Be honest and do your best to communicate mindfully
- ♥ Give 100% without expecting anything in return

- ♥ Give yourself time or space when needed to refresh yourself
- ♥ Examine your own actions and beliefs, then forgive

Consider how Dr. Suvrat Bhargave's definition of a healthy relationship could help your own relationships if each of them was *"mutually nurturing and mutually respectful"* as he teaches. *My own relationships improve when I keep this in mind.*

Forgiveness Is a Bridge

If you have built walls to protect yourself from past wounds and people who have hurt you or if you have shut yourself off because you are disappointed in yourself for past mistakes, then learning to forgive is the bridge to better relationships with yourself and others. Forgiveness is a concept that takes time to understand and has a different meaning for everyone. However, if you have closed off your heart because it is too painful to examine past events, you are closing yourself off to healing and peace of mind. Forgiving does not mean you have to enter back into a relationship with someone who has injured or abused you. It means you forgive—for you—to set yourself free from anger, resentment and thoughts of harm.

Whenever I forgive anyone, it sets me free.
~ Robert Holden, author, *Shift Happens*

Forgiveness and Healing Your Heart

We now know that heart disease and type 2 Diabetes are linked. Along with improved eating habits, being active and reducing stress, we must include the ability to love, to be loved *and* to forgive. Dean Ornish, M.D. is one of the pioneers in the field of research in reversing the plaque built up in arteries and teaching people how to prevent heart disease. He has written national bestselling books, including *8 Pathways to Intimacy and Health.* We know that intimacy improves the quality of our lives. Yet most people don't realize how much it can increase the quality of our health, happiness and survival. Dr. Ornish writes:

> I am not aware of any other factor in medicine that has a greater impact on our survival than the healing power of love and intimacy. Not diet, not smoking, not exercise, not stress, not genetics, not drugs, not surgery.

Dr. Ornish reveals that the real epidemic in modern culture is not only physical heart disease but also what he calls emotional and spiritual heart disease: loneliness, isolation, alienation and depression. He illustrates that the very defenses that we think protect us from emotional pain are often the same ones that actually heighten our pain and threaten our survival. Dr. Ornish outlines pathways to intimacy and healing – turning sadness into happiness, suffering into joy.

The Importance of Forgiveness

Forgiveness does not condone or excuse someone for their actions, rather it helps empower and free you from the pain of chronic anger, separation and isolation. It is equally as important to forgive yourself as it is the other person. Just as chronic stress can suppress your immune function, *altruism, love and compassion may enhance it*. Studies have proven that *seeing an act of kindness* produces a release of protective antibodies in our systems. Here are a few things to consider regarding forgiveness:

- ♥ Group support and confession helps us heal.
- ♥ Forgiving the abuser does not condone the abuse.
- ♥ When you can share your darkest secrets and mistakes with another person who listens without judgment, it is like shining a light in the darkness. A powerful social bond of intimacy is forged. You reintegrate those parts of yourself that may have been split off because they seemed the most painful and least lovable.
- ♥ When someone else can have compassion, forgiveness and acceptance of those dark parts of ourselves that seem so unlovable, it makes it easier for us to accept those parts within us. When we can do this, we are less likely to project our darkness onto others and hate them. If we don't acknowledge our anger, we are more prone to violence. As we have more compassion for our own weakness, it becomes easier to feel more empathy and forgiveness for the ignorance and darkness we experience in others. This experience is healing for the one asking for forgiveness as well as the other who is offering it.

> One thing you get from caring for others is that you are not lonely. And
> the more connected you are the healthier you are. ~ Dr. James Lynch

Dr. Dick Tibbits in his book, *Forgive to Live*, shares that forgiveness is not a delete button; it is not *whether you remember, but how you remember* an event. He adds, "You can forgive people and still hold them accountable for their actions. *What changes is your desire for vengeance. Forgiveness sets you free.* Forgiveness is the process of reframing one's anger and hurt from the past, with the goal of recovering one's peace in the present and revitalizing one's purpose and hopes for the future."

Forgiveness is the work you need to do for your own well-being. Dr. Dick Tibbits offers many tips for forgiveness in his books and seminars. Here are a few:

- Accept that life is not fair and others may play by a different set of rules
- Stop blaming others for your circumstances
- You cannot change the person who hurt you; you can only change yourself
- Recognize that only you can make the choice to forgive
- If you want to live, at some point you must choose to forgive

Peace starts with each one of us. When we have inner peace, we
can be at peace with those around us. ~ The Dalai Lama
An affirmation for forgiveness:

When I forgive, I heal myself and others

I could not end this chapter on relationships without mentioning that we have our own relationships with things like clutter, food, and money which can keep us trapped. Having a problem with clutter can mean anything from lacking organizational skills, to just having too much stuff, to hanging onto things for security. Having issues with food can mean that we don't value ourselves enough to take care of our bodies. We may overeat out of fear and need for comfort. Our relationship with money can stem from the way we were raised, or simply lacking information on how to handle finances. Whatever your relationship is with clutter, food or money, know that you have the power to change your beliefs and behaviors. At the end of this chapter are resources that will not only change your relationships, but will empower you to improve your life.

Where do you *want to start changing your relationships? Who do you need to spend more quality time with? How will you make changes?*

♥ **Health Coach Wisdom:** In the Tecumseh Community Health Study, investigators found that activities involving regular volunteer work were among the most powerful predictors of mortality rates. Those who volunteered to help others at least once a week were two and a half times *less likely* to die. In other words, those who helped others helped themselves.

Action step:

Complete this exercise to help improve your relationships. *Begin by taking action with journaling, taking a relationship course, reading a book or seeing a counselor.*

The top five things I would like to do to improve my relationships are:

1. _____
2. _____
3. _____
4. _____
5. _____

Marriage is a partnership and couples can't win with money
unless they're doing the budget as a team.
~Dave Ramsey, Radio host and author *Financial Peace*

Following are some resources that may help you on your journey to well-being:

Counselors, family therapists or social workers can help you learn ways to deal with conflict, manage anger and control stress. To find a therapist, psychiatrist or therapy group visit www. Psycologytoday.com, or www.therapistlocator.net – a public service of the American Association for Marriage and Family Therapy.

Employee assistance programs (EAP's) may offer referrals to counseling to help employees with issues like alcohol, drugs, job stress and relationships.

If you have problems with alcohol or drugs call the Center or Substance Abuse Treatment's Referral Service at 1800-662-HELP (4357). Or visit www.aa.org for support.

If someone you care about has addiction problems go to www.al-anon.alateen.org for alcohol or www.nar-anon.org for drug addiction to get support for yourself.

Peter Walsh, www.peterwalshdesign.com: Peter Walsh, author, "Enough Already", books, DVDs and advice on clearing clutter from your life.

Dorthy Breininger, www.dorthytheorganizer.com: Helping you control your clutter.

Dave Ramsey, www.daveramsey.com: books and resources you need to start your journey to financial peace from American Financial author and radio host.

Suze Orman, www.suzeorman.com. Take charge of your personal finances with author and financial expert Suze's tools: books, audio programs and more.

Katie and Gay Hendricks, www.hendricks.com: Secrets to creating easy, lasting love.

Between stimulus and response there is a space. In that space is our power to
choose our response. In our response lies our growth and our freedom.
~Viktor E. Frankl, Psychiatrist, holocaust survivor
and author of *Man's Search for Meaning*

Books and resources

Love and Survival: 8 Pathways to Intimacy and Health by Dean Ornish, *1999*

Forgive to Live: How Forgiveness Can Save Your Life by Dr. Dick Tibbits, 2008.

Loveability-Knowing How to Love and Be Loved, by Robert Holden, Ph.D. 2013

Nonviolent Communication, by Marshall B. Rosenberg, Ph.D. Life-Changing Tools for Healthy Relationships, 2003.

How to Win Friends and Influence People and *The 5 Essential People Skills- How to Assert Yourself, Listen to Others and Resolve Conflicts,* Dale Carnegie Training, Simon & Schuster, 1998.

The Power of Kindness: The Unexpected Benefits of Leading a Compassionate Life by Piero Ferruci, Penguin group, New York, 2007.

Emotional Freedom by Dr. Judith Orloff, M.D. 2010, or visit www.drjudithorloff.com

To find out more about relationship coaching:

- www.JackCanfield.com. The Success Principles Coaching Programs
- www.anthonyrobbins.com. Anthony Robbins.
- www.alancohen.com, Alan Cohen.
- www.hendricks.com. Gay and Katie Hendricks International Learning Center teaches core relationship skills.

For more information about wellness coaching: www.lynellross.com

Chapter 5
Reduce Stress and Live a Joyful Life

People are disturbed not by a thing, but by their perception of a thing.

~Epictetus

It is impossible to be stressed out and joyful at the same time. How much time do you spend being stressed out rather than joyful? What does being joy mean to you? Taking time to learn about stress can help you reduce it and become happier and healthier.

The research that I've done on stress focuses on reducing or coping with stress. This chapter contains many tips to accomplish that. Additionally, I would like to offer a revolutionary idea for you to consider. What if you could set the goal to *eliminate stress?* Most people would say that's impossible. However, *if we get what we think about,* and we set the bar too low by thinking we have to live with stress, then our lives will be stressful. Personally, I've decided that I don't want to have a stressful life and I've learned that most of my stress was created by me! I either put too much pressure on myself or I didn't realize that *I can control my thoughts* about what is happening. I know that I have no control over the weather, disasters, aging, death, taxes and other people, but I have the ability to *question my thoughts about these things.* The more successful I am in learning to cope with life's events, the less stress I will have. If my goal is to eliminate or reduce stress, I must believe I can do it. I can and so can you.

Life is moving at a fast pace these days. Technology is changing at staggering speeds. Just when we learn how to use our newest smart phone, software program or computer, a new model comes out and we have to learn something new to keep up. Families are busier than ever, kid's schedules are so full that there isn't a minute of downtime, and most people don't know what it is like to live in a peaceful environment.

It is possible to manage your busy schedule and create the life you want. After all, *it is your life.* The first step is in understanding what you want, what you don't want, what you value most, and who matters most to you. If you take time for planning and reflection, you will see things more clearly. If you are moving at breakneck speed you may be unconsciously working for things *because the ideas have been marketed to you.*

Advertising is designed to make you want things out of fear. The constantly flashing images of expensive cars, beautiful people in designer clothes, drinking and eating rich foods, tempt you to think you aren't enough without them. But what good is it to rush and stress over obtaining things if we don't have time to enjoy them? Usually, once we purchase that new item, we still feel empty. No amount of material things will ever make you happy.

There is a way to have what you desire and still be able to enjoy your life with the people you love. Decide what you value most, and make a plan to concentrate on things that are your highest priority. The key is to let go and spend less time on the things that are draining your energy or hurting you. You detach from wanting more when you stop trying to prove yourself. You are good enough already.

When I help clients prioritize their values they do well until a crisis happens. Then they postpone coaching appointments and stop taking care of themselves. That is when routine habits and a coach or trusted friend are most important. Stress is manageable if you understand what it is, where it comes from and when you have strategies in place to deal with it. Take good care yourself during stressful times and you will think more clearly and handle problems more effectively. *The better care you take of your physical and mental health, the fewer problems you will have.*

What is Stress?

Stress is a mental tension and worry caused by problems in your life, work and surroundings. Stress causes you worry and anxiety. Symptoms are pressure, nervous, worry, anxiety, trouble, difficulty.

There are three types of stress:

Acute Stress: Fight, flight or freeze. A threat is perceived. The body prepares to defend itself. The autonomic nervous system automatically puts the body on alert. The adrenal cortex automatically releases hormones which makes the heart beat harder and more rapidly. Breathing automatically becomes more rapid. The thyroid gland automatically stimulates the metabolism, and the larger muscles receive more oxygenated blood. It takes about ninety minutes for the metabolism to return to normal when the response is over. The part of the brain that initiates the flight or fight response, the amygdale, cannot distinguish between a real threat and a perceived threat. *Sometimes the perceived threat is so intense it triggers a "freeze" response.* Our brain gets overwhelmed by a threat causing our muscles to get tense and ready for action. When we stay in the state, the result is often stiffness and knots in our backs, shoulders, neck, jaw and arms.

Chronic Stress: This is the constant pressures of daily living such as financial worries, parenting issues, job concerns, or your critical boss. This is the stress we tend to ignore or suppress. Left uncontrolled, this stress affects your health, your body and your immune system. Dr. Joel Dimsdale of UC, San Diego, wrote in the Journal of the American College of Cardiology, "There is overwhelming evidence that stress creates an environment where heart attacks and even sudden death become more likely."

Eustress: This is good stress that has positive connotations. Stress can be helpful and good when it motivates us to do more. Graduating, getting married, having a baby, getting a promotion and winning money can be causes of Eustress.

What *Causes* Stress?

Awareness is the key to coping with stress. Identifying and making a plan to handle it are your best defenses. These are common causes of stress:

- Relationships
- Health Issues
- Death of a loved one
- Time management
- Work
- Finances
- Overloaded schedule

Stress can also be caused from not knowing what you want, not having a plan, not following through, or not knowing what your values and priorities are. Stress is also caused by fear and many things that we face daily such as:

- Not speaking up for ourselves and not having boundaries
- Believing our negative or stressful thoughts
- Not knowing what our needs are
- Neglecting our bodies and pushing ourselves too hard
- Taking ourselves too seriously
- Our ego telling us we aren't good enough
- Blaming others for our feelings and our troubles
- Change: divorce, death, lack of money, loss of job, moving
- Wanting more, by never being satisfied

- Rushing
- Our attitude about aging
- Being overweight and overeating
- Fear of not trusting yourself
- Clutter and buying things we don't need
- Trying to make changes too fast or all at once

As you learn to stop arguing with reality, let go of trying to control what's outside of your control, and start making clear choices about how you want to be and behave in the world, you'll find yourself with less stress and greater serenity than ever before.
~ Michael Neill, Author of *Feel Happy Now!*

What Does Stress Do to Us?

According to The Mayo Clinic in Rochester, Minnesota, here are just a few of the effects stress has on your body: Headache, chest pain, pounding heart, high blood pressure, muscle aches, grinding teeth, clinched jaws, indigestion, constipation, diarrhea, stomach cramping or bloating, fatigue, insomnia, weight gain or weight loss. *Stress also contributes to heart disease*, skin conditions and certain cancers by weakening the immune system.

The effects of stress on your thoughts and feelings: Excessive worrying, anxiety, anger, irritability, depression, sadness, restlessness, mood swings, feeling insecure, confusion, resentment, forgetfulness, blaming others, guilt and more.

The effects of stress on your behavior: Overeating, loss of appetite, angry outbursts, crying spells, burnout, change in sleep nervous twitch, impatience and more.

Seven Keys to Stop Emotional Stress

1. **Improve Your Relationships by Setting Boundaries**
   In the previous chapter we looked at ways to be more open and less judgmental. When you make your relationships a priority, you will significantly reduce your stress level. However, as we have all experienced, relationships cause some of our most challenging stressors. Some people are just difficult, yet sometimes it is our inability to relate to others that causes many of our problems. In order to significantly reduce your stress you must know your standards, set boundaries and be able to say *no*.

   When you know what your standards are, *those things you hold yourself to*, you will be centered and not so easily swayed. Boundaries *are those things you hold to prevent others from impacting you*. Personal boundaries are like imaginary lines created to protect us from the damaging behavior of others. Boundaries are necessary to keep unwanted behaviors from negatively affecting your well-being and they help you to make better choices. Here are the steps to take in setting boundaries:

- **Identify the behaviors that are not acceptable to you**: For example: *People may not hit me, yell at me, manipulate me or try to make me feel guilty. I will not listen to gossip or allow people to smoke in my home.*
- **Explain to others what is unacceptable**: Calmly inform the person what you won't tolerate. For example, *"You are criticizing me and it is hurtful to me."*
- **Make a request**: Let others know what is acceptable. *"Please do not yell at me."*
- **Give a warning**: Let the other person know what you will do if they continue. *"If you continue yelling, I will leave the room."*
- **Follow through**: It is crucial that you follow through with the stated consequence if the person ignores you. *"What you are doing is unacceptable, so I'm leaving."*
- **Learn to say no and understand the guilty feelings**: You have a right to say no without explaining why. You need be able to say no and feel the uncomfortable feelings. Saying no is often crucial to your well-being.
- **Let it go**: Once you've stated what is acceptable and have taken action, let go of what happens. Their behavior is not about you and you cannot manage other people's perceptions and feelings.

Asking and expecting others to treat you appropriately is a necessary step
in learning to take care of yourself and it allows you to develop healthy
relationships, exhibit self-respect and become a role-model for others.
~*The Wellcoaches® Coaching Psychology Manual*

2. **Change Your Self-Talk**
You have the power to change your thoughts, *but first you have to notice what you are saying to yourself.* The automatic thoughts that run through your head can be mostly negative, causing you to have a more pessimistic outlook. Conversely, if your thoughts are mostly positive, you are more of an optimist. Studies show that your way of thinking affects your quality of life. This is your explanatory style. Being optimistic helps you to cope with stressful situations, reducing stressful effects.

Is It True?
Byron Katie is an author who teaches a method of self-inquiry known as "The Work of Byron Katie." The Work is a way of questioning and identifying any stressful thought. It consists of four questions and a turn around. *The four questions are: 1) Is it true? 2)*

Can you absolutely know that it is true? 3) How do you react, what happens, when you believe that thought? 4) Who would you be without the thought? The turnaround involves considering the thought in reverse form. The Work is a way of identifying and questioning the thoughts that cause anger, fear, depression, addiction and violence. Through Byron Katie's Work thousands of people have experienced happiness through undoing these negative, fearful thoughts and allowing their minds to return to its true, awakened, peaceful, nature. *For more information see the resources at the end of this chapter.*

> By actively exercising kindness and appreciation, we can promote
> the brain's natural production of oxytocin and dopamine, two
> chemicals that help us feel pleasure and well being.
> ~ Dr. Linda Miles, *Mindfulness as a Path to Joy and Healing*

Below are some ways that we develop irrational thinking. Instead, develop the habit of a positive alternative.

All or nothing thinking: We see things as all bad instead of *focusing on the things we did well.* We only hear the critical comments and not the compliments.

Catastrophizing: We make things more important than they are, or *anticipate the worst happening* instead of thinking: *"I'll plan for the worst, but expect the best."*

Perfectionist: When we think everything has to be perfect or that we have to do everything right. When we see things as good or bad with no room for in between, we create unnecessary stress for ourselves. *Strive for progress, not perfection.*

We take things personally: If things don't go well, we assume it is our fault. We blame ourselves or hear what others say as negative by assuming the worst. *Become your own best friend and stand by yourself no matter what.*

3. **Stand up to Fear**
   I have attended many seminars related to the brain and how we think, and have read many books illuminating the difference between our lower self (ego) and our higher self (unconditioned self). There are different names for these two opposites, but one thing is very obvious to me, that when we think from our higher self, we are calm, wise and clear.
   One of these sources of information came from Susan Jeffers, PhD, in her book *Feel the Fear and Do It Anyway.* Jeffers points out that stress comes from fear. There are three levels of fear. Level one fears are things like making decisions, changing a career,

dying, illness, losing weight, ending or beginning a relationship, public speaking and making a mistake. Level two fears are failure, rejection, being vulnerable, loss of image or being conned. The level three fear is "I can't handle it." Jeffers explains: *"At the bottom of every one of your fears is simply the fear that you can't handle whatever life may bring you."* In *Feel the Fear and Do It Anyway and Feel the Fear and Beyond,* Jeffers teaches truths for handling your fears. "If you knew that you could handle anything that came your way, what would you possibly have to fear? The answer is nothing!"

This next principle has helped me to overcome my fears. From her teachings I learned that I have no control over what happens to anything outside myself. I have no control over my spouse, my friends, my family or the world. According to Jeffers, here is the secret to stopping our worries:

All you have to do to diminish your fear is to develop more trust in your ability to handle whatever comes your way!

The strategy I developed is to learn to trust and forgive myself. When I trust myself to react appropriately in any situation I don't have to fear what others do. If I make a mistake and I forgive myself, I learn from the mistake and have grown.

4. **Embrace Spirituality**
Developing a spiritual practice has been shown to reduce stress and contribute to a healthier, happier life. Through my research of spiritual masters, psychologists and enlightened seekers, I learned that being joyful is our true nature.

5. **Allow Acceptance**
Accepting *what is* will help you to avoid being hurt, frustrated and angry more than any concept you can master. Reflect on the wisdom of the Serenity Prayer:

> *God grant me the serenity to accept*
> *The things I cannot change,*
> *Courage to change the things I can*
> *And the wisdom to know the difference.*

6. **Avoid Trouble**
If you want a peaceful, stress-free life, look ahead to the situations, people and possible sources of drama that may upset you. Be prepared by noticing things that may trigger negative emotions. Remove yourself from difficult situations. Byron Katie, Author of *Loving What Is* says, *"When your mind is on someone else's business, no one is doing your job."* In other words *avoid drama and focus on what you need to do.*

If you are the person that people call when they get into trouble, make an effort to notice if you attract drama by being the one that "fixes" everyone's problems. If you take time to examine this habit, you may find that you are not really helping, just draining your own energy. When people unload troubles on you, they feel better temporarily while you feel exhausted, knowing you didn't solve anything. Carolyn Myss, PhD, spiritual leader and author of many books including "Why People Don't Heal and How They Can" taught me how to avoid getting involved in other's problems. I heard Carolyn's advice to a caller on her Hay House Radio program where she told a woman to offer loving support while staying detached. "People know what is best for themselves," said Myss. This advice hit home with me and cured me of my need to "fix things" for others. I appreciate the wise counsel of Carolyn Myss.

7. **Embrace Change**
One of the greatest stressors for many people is change, and *it is certain*. Just when you think you have landed your dream job, you get laid off. When you think you have everything under control, you get the phone call that someone you love is getting a divorce or has had an accident. Change happens daily. Keeping an open mind to handle any new situation will help you feel stronger and happier. If you haven't had successes to draw from, then you might not have an optimistic view. In spite of this, *it is possible to change your habits and beliefs.* If you have faith in yourself, you can make positive changes and create a better situation.

> Progress is impossible without change, and those who cannot
> change their mind cannot change anything.
> ~ George Bernard Shaw

Physical Strategies for Managing Stress

Meditate. Meditation has been proven to change your brain. Rebecca Gladding co-author of *You Are Not Your Brain*, clinical instructor and attending psychiatrist at UCLA, explains how your brain changes when you mediate. "Sitting to meditate every day for at least fifteen to thirty minutes makes a huge difference in how you approach life, how personally you take things and how you interact with others. It enhances compassion, allows you to see more clearly, including yourself and creates a sense of calm." In a recent article for Psychology Today, she further explained the science behind how the different parts of the brain are responsible for allowing us to process information, change habits and feel empathy. When we meditate we are able to see ourselves and everyone around us from a clearer perspective, while simultaneously being more present, compassionate and empathetic with people no matter what the situation.

Beginning Meditation

Get quiet somewhere so you can begin to calm down. If you do not already have a prayer or meditation practice you can seek help through your church, through yoga or meditation teachers, on-line classes and books. From the writings of Sri Chinmoy's *Guide to Healthy and Happy Living*, he describes one kind of meditation:

> *If you want peace, then you have to meditate on peace. If you want love, then you have to meditate on love. If you want joy or any other divine quality, the best thing is to meditate on it. Each individual will have a different way of meditating. It is important to keep the spine straight and the body relaxed. Close your eyes and go within, focusing your conscious attention both on the physical plane and the subconscious plane.*

Many different types of meditation techniques can calm your mind and reduce stress. When you first learn to meditate, your thoughts may be as distracting as billboards racing by on a highway. Let them run. Those thoughts are your lower self, your ego thoughts. Your mind will stop spinning and will begin to get quiet. As you sit, your inner world becomes clear and calm. When your thoughts relax you will experience stillness until you begin to hear the "still small voice within", your higher self. That is the treasure and where peace and all your answers are found.

Here is a simple meditation technique to start with:

- ♥   Get comfortable, wear comfortable clothing.
- ♥   Sit in a quiet place with no interruptions.
- ♥   Relax your muscles from head to toe
- ♥   Close your eyes and focus on your breath
- ♥   Repeat one phrase such as "I am calm or I am peaceful."

Author Louise Hay suggests meditating on the question:

"What is it that I need to know?"

More tips for managing stress:

Organize your day. Each day, make a list of things to do and categorize by priority. Be careful not to put too many things on your list. Break them into groups of A, B and C. If you are feeling overwhelmed, only do the things that have to get done this day. Writing down what to do takes the confusion out of your head and releases it on paper.

Look back at your list. What things do you need to let go of? What commitments can you drop to relieve stress? Be brutal. Your self-care should come first.

Make time each day to relax and do something you enjoy. This is especially true for hard driving personalities. Get a massage or walk outside. It is not only important to relax, it is vital to your well-being. It will re-vitalize and give you a new perspective.

Eat nutritious brain foods. Your food affects your mood. Eat foods high in B vitamins such as whole grains, cereals and brown rice. Foods high in antioxidants combat stress, such as dark green vegetables, fresh fruits with vitamin C, oranges, tangerines, and sweet peppers. Lean proteins such as beef, chicken, fish, nuts, protein powder and peanut butter feed your brain. The amino acids in these foods are high in protein and are the key to helping you feel happier. Eating from the food groups will keep your energy high, your immune system healthy and your brain balanced and calm.

Eat breakfast. Your mind and body cannot function on an empty stomach and your energy and mood will drop by early morning if you skip breakfast.

Hydrate with water: Your brain is made up of mostly water and needs approximately sixty-four ounces per day to keep you fresh and thinking clearly.

Move: Get up and move or walk for five minutes out of every fifty-five to circulate the oxygen in your blood up to your brain. Moving transforms stress and overwhelm into positive energy. Getting some sunshine which makes Vitamin D is vital to our health, so getting outside provides additional motivation to move.

Breathe Deeply: When you find yourself stressed, overwhelmed or holding your breathe-stop and inhale deeply filling your lungs, then slowly exhale.

Close your eyes. Rest your eyes every twenty minutes from your computer. When you shut your eye lids for 1 minute you calm down your brain and can refocus. If meditating is not possible, then take a five minute break to close your eyes and sort things out. Let worries fall away. Connect to your higher self.

Let go. View your mistakes as learning opportunities not as failures.

Talk to a trusted friend, counselor or mentor. Discussing your concerns with a supportive person frees your mind.

Break a big goal into small steps. Change is much easier and you are more likely to succeed if you break your goal down into small steps and proceed one step at a time. Focus on the task and don't jump ahead. With each task you accomplish, your stress level goes down and your self-esteem rises.

Use affirmations. Using affirmations helps you build yourself up and make changes. Write a positive statement making sure to write it as if it is already happening: *I handle anything that comes my way.*

Remember, this too shall pass. Nothing lasts forever. You will get through this difficult time. Just say to yourself, whatever happens: *Everything works out for my highest good.*

Three Actions Steps to Help You Get Started:

1. **Get Organized:** Identify your stressors. Decide what you can let go of or change. Are you putting too many demands on yourself? Are you willing to ask for help? Make a list of responsibilities, then sort your list by things that must be done and the things that you are demanding of yourself. What can you take off the list?
2. **Be Realistic:** There are only so many hours in the day. Make time work for you. To fit in healthy habits such as exercise and eating well, you may have to let go of certain obligations. Be honest with yourself. What are you doing in order to avoid doing undesirable tasks like paying bills, exercising or clearing clutter? Consider getting help from a mental health professional or health coach. Seeking help is a wise choice as these professionals can help you to see things from a new perspective and can help you move forward if you feel overwhelmed.
3. **Put your health on your list:** The secret to good health is fitting healthy habits into your daily life. Make a list of the healthy habits that make you feel better and fit them into your daily schedule. Decide how you are going to drink, eat, sleep, move and interact with other people each day. Make choices that work for you rather than against your health. What you tell yourself about every choice will make it difficult or easy, depending on your perception. *For a sample daily health schedule, visit my website at www.lynellross.com.*

Retrain Your Brain from Stress to Joy

Turn off the television. Cast aside the magazines.
These will teach you nothing of the love at the heart of you,
nothing of your soul. Now go outside into the divine world.
Breathe in the dancing air; drink in the colors and sounds.
Every leaf and cloud is a billboard for the infinite energy of living.
~ Ingrid Goff-Maidoff, *Befriending the Soul*

Most stress is an imagined state, something we create for ourselves. Losing your job or going through a divorce are very real stress factors. However, it is your thoughts about the problem make your stress level worse. The greater the stress level, the more irrational your thoughts become.

One thing that I do to relieve my stress is to listen to Hay House Radio. It was started by Louise Hay, who created it to be "radio for your soul." I always learn something new about wellness when I listen. One morning I was listening to Dr. Christiane Northrup, M.D., bestselling author and host of Flourish on Hay House Radio. She featured Dr. Laurel Mellin on her program, author of *Wired for Joy, Emotional Brain Training.* "Imagine training your emotional brain for optimal fitness. You can't think your way out of a negative emotional state," Dr. Mellin said." You can only change your emotional state in the present moment. When the stress hits, you can use tools to take you to a different brain state," according to Dr. Mellin. She believes our natural state is joy and she has created a program that gives you the power to take control of your emotions to bring you back to your natural brain state of joy.

Dr. Mellin teaches that our brains can't be in stress and joy at the same time. When we are in a state of stress, our brain naturally demands joy and will seek out sources of joy such as sugary foods and other artificial substitutes that can even become addictive. Her program works by helping you to access the lower part of the brain, the emotional part, which is very powerful. *Most of our brains are in the habit of being in stress, which causes 80% of our health problems.* When you are able to trace the source of your stress, frustration, and anger, back to fear or sadness, the process helps you transfer that stress to more rational thoughts and emotions like gratitude, happiness, security and joy.

♥ **Health Coach Wisdom:** People who are in a class, group or who seek help from a trusted person, have much greater success than by trying to reduce help alone.

Make a list of five things that cause you stress and *how you will handle them:*

1. _____
2. _____
3. _____
4. _____
5. _____

Be happy. It is one way of being wise.
~Sidonie Gabrielle Colette

A technique I use for sorting out life's problems is My Filing Cabinet Tool. Try it:

Instructions for "My Filing Cabinet" Tool:

Identify all areas of your life where you feel you have responsibilities or concerns. Place each item in a category. Each person or item will have its own "folder" (a separate line on paper). We cannot think about two things at once. When we are overwhelmed and thoughts tumble around in our head, we are not giving ourselves a chance to solve problems, only to worry. In order to gain new perspective, write down and put each item away in its "file folder" in your cabinet or until you have time to focus on only that item.

My Filing Cabinet of Life's Responsibilities: *Tool for Reducing Stress*

📁 Life Area	Concern	Concern
📁 My Health		
📁 My Family		
📁 My Friends		
📁 My Finances		
📁 My Career/Job		
📁 My Personal Growth or Spirituality		
📁 My Nutrition / Energy		
📁 My Sense of Purpose		
📁 My Fitness		
📁 My Sleep		
📁 My House/ Office		

♥ **Health Coach Wisdom:** Often your solution comes after you've had a chance to focus on it, *and then put it away.*

I keep this list by my computer where I see it daily to help me stay centered:

Today May I

- ♥ Expand my awareness
- ♥ Make a plan for today which reduces my stress
- ♥ Build healthy habits
- ♥ Manage what I focus on—seeing the good in everything
- ♥ Keep working toward my goals
- ♥ Bring kindness to every situation
- ♥ Move from surviving to thriving
- ♥ Think and act from my higher self in each moment

Moving From Stress to Joy

Wherever you go, carry happiness with you. ~Sri Chinmoy

Having fun and experiencing joy are among the secrets to wellness. In my life I had not taken much time for fun or play; I was too busy taking care of things on my "To Do" lists. I made sure my kids, friends and relatives had fun, but it wasn't something I'd take time for.

I was fortunate enough to attend a five day coaching training by Dr. Robert Holden, one of the most positive and innovative leaders on our planet today. His work on positive psychology and spirituality has been featured on programs from PBS to Oprah. He founded the Happiness Project and has written many best-selling books including Loveability and Happiness Now! Among his corporate clients is Dove and the "Real Beauty Campaign. What drew me to the training was the title: Coaching Happiness.

What made the training was the teacher. I have never met a kinder, more approachable, funnier or more genuine person than Robert Holden. I have certifications from areas of wellness: nutrition, fitness, life coaching, lifestyle coaching, etc. Yet prior to this training, something was missing. I have achieved almost every goal I have ever set—yet I had forgotten what happiness was. I spent my entire life making lists and reaching goals, but in the process of working so hard, I had forgotten how to play and I always felt an underlying uneasiness. After spending five days with a group of like-minded people participating in workshop activities with Robert, I came away a changed person. I participated earnestly, absorbing Robert's inspirational teachings. I understood what was missing–giving myself permission to be happy and realizing that I have the power to be happy now, not when I have achieved something. When it was over I knew that I would have to practice to integrate what I had learned. I also had to do some "forgiveness work."

Ironically, my mother and relatives had always told me that I was an easy going child, a good girl. I learned to be a people-pleaser. When I was a senior in high school, what I wrote next to my yearbook picture was "The most important thing in life is being happy." Ouch. Years later when I re-read that in my yearbook I was embarrassed of my simple mindedness and hoped no one had seen it. However, by the end of the workshop I realized I had been very smart for a seventeen year old. My big take-away lesson from the Happiness Coaching Training was that the most important thing is to be happy. If we are happy and love ourselves then we will be loving toward others and inspired to make contributions to the world. I learned how important it is to forgive myself and others, and to believe that I we have a right to be happy. Before I left for the training, I was embarrassed to tell people where I was going, fearing they might think it was silly. It turned out to be the most important education I have ever received. Dr. Holden graciously teaches that we have our "ego self," and we have our "unconditioned or true self." The highest part of us is peaceful, loving, kind and wise. If only we all connected with our higher self more, what a peaceful and loving world we would live in. Information on Robert Holden's resources are listed at the end of this chapter.

> People who follow their joy discover a depth of creativity
> and talent that inspires the world.
> ~ Dr. Robert Holden

When you have some quiet moments, please consider reflecting on the following questions: How happy are you? How happy do you allow yourself to be? How deserving do you think you are? What is happiness to you?

We are more wired to focus on the negative than the positive and we don't do very well at recognizing or feeling our emotions. Thanks to the work of people like Dr. Martin E. P.

Seligman, we are learning more about groundbreaking scientific research that shows how positive psychology is shifting from mental illness to positive emotion. Happiness, studies show, is not the result of good genes or luck. It can be cultivated by identifying and nurturing traits that we already possess, including kindness, humor, optimism and generosity. In his books *Authentic Happiness* and *Learned Optimism*, Seligman offers examples and exercises to identify your strengths, boost your immune system and make you happier:

> Anytime you find yourself down, anxious or angry, ask what you are saying to yourself. Sometimes the beliefs will turn out to be accurate; when this is so, concentrate on ways you can alter the situation and prevent adversity from becoming a disaster. But usually your negative beliefs are distortions. Challenge them. Don't let them run your emotional life. Once you get into the habit of disputing negative beliefs, your daily life will run much better, and you will feel much happier.

> It is Joy that I wish you above all else.
> Joy found through love, silence, play and laughter.
> Joy found through knowing who you really are.
> ~ Ingrid Goff-Maidoff, author, poet

♥ **Health Coach Wisdom:** Every morning ask yourself, "How happy will I allow myself to be today?"

Happiness is a Choice

Author, speaker and life coach Michael Neill offers a way to see happiness in a new light. I've seen Michael speak in person, listened to his radio program, read his books and was a student of his "*Impossible Goal*" class. His guidance and insights were the catalyst I needed to turn the dream of this book into reality. He has a unique quality of being able to provoke new insights and a clarity which leave you feeling better instantly. From my viewpoint, he helps you become happier by teaching you how to feel more of your good feelings and becoming more comfortable with your difficult ones.

Candace Pert, PhD was a neuroscientist who wrote the foreword for Michael Neill's book, *Feel Happy Now!* She also helped discover a fundamental element of brain chemistry and went on to become a major proponent of alternative medicine and of the unity of mind and body, *the ability of emotions to affect health.* "I've come to believe that virtually all illness, if not psychosomatic in foundation, has a definite psychosomatic component. Our culture has been drugging the brain to alter its chemistry and unrealistically overemphasized in terms of the role it plays in controlling our moods."

She wrote, "Now that taking drugs has replaced working on yourself and your life, and now that anti-anxiety and anti depressant medications can be prescribed by any type of physician, the lack of counseling and sensitivity to the power of consciousness as a healing force has become endemic...Michael Neill steps forward in this book as a powerful spokesman for the wonderful world of the mind."

Through his coaching Michael Neill encourages you to be happy because it feels good, it makes you healthier and "it makes you younger."

Happiness leads to success a lot more often than success leads to happiness.
~ Michael Neill

What is Joy for You?

I reached out to people asking what they do for "fun." I received marvelous responses:

- We bike. It's a good way to travel and see the country. Then we reward ourselves with ice cream. You can do that when you cycle 80 miles!
- Spending time with family and friends especially when there's lots of laughter.
- Just taking in the natural beauty all around us makes me happy. Counting my blessings also makes me feel appreciative, content and happy.
- Being cute. I love looking good 24/7! (*hairdresser and fashionista*)
- I love watching the trees start to bloom and my bulbs bring forth color. Sharing beautiful sunsets with my friends.
- Going to a wonderful music concert with a good friend.

If you never did you should
These things are fun and fun is good. ~ Dr. Seuss

I have spent my life wondering what makes people happy, but this "Joy" thing threw me. Joy seemed too big of a word for me, yet finally I understood it. To be truly joyful we must live with a fully open heart. We must be vulnerable to loss, pain and humiliation. If we numb ourselves, we may block the pain, but we will also block the pleasure. We need to spend more time doing things we love to do. We can create more happiness and positivity in our lives. What steps can we take to more joy to our lives? We can appreciate the little things. Here are a few ideas that bring joy to my life:

- ❤ Meeting my best friends to take a walk and connect from the heart
- ❤ Preparing a meal to share with loved ones or someone in need
- ❤ Spending time hiking in nature and soaking up the smell of pine trees, mountain air or the ocean. Looking up at the sky.
- ❤ Seeing my sons and family members enjoying their lives
- ❤ Picking flowers and making colorful arrangements to share with friends.
- ❤ Witnessing acts of kindness
- ❤ Sending cards and letters that may brighten someone's day
- ❤ Experiencing each moment from a grateful perspective
- ❤ Petting my dog
- ❤ Traveling and exploring new places with my husband

I have chosen to be happy
because it is good for my health.
~ Voltaire

Action Step:

Make a list of 10 things you love to do. ***Put the list where you will see it and do something you love everyday!***

1. _____
2. _____
3. _____
4. _____
5. _____
6. _____
7. _____
8. _____
9. _____
10. _____

Books & Resources:

Robert Holden, PhD, *www.robertholden.org, resources on courses, happiness tests and more. Some of Robert's book include: Happiness Now, Authentic Success,* Hay House Inc. 2007.

Feel the Fear and Do It Anyway, by Susan Jeffers, PhD. Ballantine, 2007. Visit www.susanjeffers. com for more books and audio books for more ways to build your confidence and peace of mind.

Befriending the Soul by Ingrid Goff-Maidoff. Visit her website www.TendingJoy.com for more handmade books, soul wisdom and handmade gifts.

Feel Happy Now! By Michael Neill, 2008, Hay House, Inc. www.supercoach.com

The Art of Extreme Self-Care by Cheryl Richardson, Hay House, Inc., 2009, for tips on ways to make your self-care a priority.

Everything You Need To Know To Feel Go(o)d, Candace B. Pert, PhD with Nancy Marriott.

The Joy Diet, 10 Daily Practices for a Happier Life by Martha Beck, 2003, Crown Publishers.

All is Well-Heal Your Body with Medicine, Affirmations, and Intuition, by Louise L. Hay and Mona Lisa Schultz, Hay House, Inc. 2013.

www.davidji.com. Author of *Secrets of Meditation* makes the science of meditation easy.

The Mindfulness Meditation Institute, www.MindfulnessMeditationInstitute.org

National Institute of Mental Health, www.mentalhealth.gov.

www.chopracentermeditation.com. Guided meditation Cds make learning to meditate easy.

Chapter 6
Where Personal Growth Meets Spirituality

You have believed that your health is a function of your body, but we say to you now: Look deeper. There is no aspect of your experience that is unrelated to Spirit.
~Alan Cohen, *The Dragon Doesn't Live Here Anymore*

Studying health and wellness has been a long journey for me. I learned that our thoughts direct the course of our lives, but finally realized that our command center is our heart, not our head. We must learn how to be still and listen if we are to be at peace. This did not become clear to me until I embraced spirituality.

What follows is my best interpretation of the importance of spirituality and its effect on our well-being. It is based on the teachings of spiritual masters, mentors, psychologists, life coaches and authors who have guided me on my journey. My interpretation is not meant to offend, only to offer some insights that might help you heal from pain and the frustration of daily living.

I have always loved self-help books, and read enough during the early part of my life to set me on a positive path. In the past fifteen years, I have purchased enough personal development books to build my own lending library. While researching the keys of wellness, I found that being a life-long learner contributes greatly to our health. Learning new things keeps us young, gives us something to look forward to, gives our lives greater meaning and makes things easier. Taking a class, developing a new hobby, traveling, reading new books, gardening, cooking or doing anything to expand your creativity will help you to grow and enhance your life. However, it takes courage to learn about yourself, to determine your values and examine your beliefs. The way we react to life's difficulties can be improved through the help of classes, coaches and trusted support people. A true secret to learning more about yourself is through spirituality. *Now for the hard part...*

What is Spirituality?

I went in search of answers to this question with an open mind. Following are insights I experienced on my path, the most profound is that we are more loving, powerful and joyful when we experience a spiritual connection. I had a sense that spirituality is different than religion. To me, religion seems to be man's interpretation, while spirituality is a universal understanding that we are connected to something beyond words. As a result, it is possible to be religious without being spiritual, to be spiritual without being religious, or to have a combination of both. In my quest for spiritual understanding, I found that love, appreciation, kindness, service, wonder, peace and compassion are among the common concepts associated with spirituality. These are possible when we are living fully in the present moment.

> Constantly apply cheerfulness, if for no other reason than because you
> are on this spiritual path. Have a sense of gratitude to everything, even
> difficult emotions, because of their potential to wake you up.
> ~Pema Chödrön

The question was asked of Rabbi Rami Shapiro, award winning author, poet and teacher, "I'm not religious, and I don't believe in God, but I am spiritual. Does spirituality require believing in God?" His reply:

> No, but it does require you to think these things through. For me, God is
> the source and substance of all life; religious means belonging to a specific
> religion and conforming to its rules and teachings; and spiritual means
> cultivating an ever-greater awareness of the sanctity of all life, leading to
> an ever-greater commitment to justice, gratitude and compassion for all life.

The always eloquent Marianne Williamson, internationally acclaimed author and lecturer is a premier authority on spirituality. I have admired her for many years, attended her lectures and read some of her later books, but it wasn't until I read *A Return to Love* that spirituality made sense to me. *A Return to Love* is based on Marianne's interpretation and reflections on *A Course in Miracles*. I kept hearing of it, but resisted reading it fearing that I wouldn't be able to interpret it. I didn't have to; Marianne Williamson has done this brilliantly for us. If you have any desire to heal from emotional or physical pain, from trauma or sadness, *A Return to Love* will bring you comfort. I knew it was going to reveal spiritual secrets when I read it. Marianne teaches:

> A miracle is a shift in perception from fear to love.

As she carefully lays the framework for spirituality, what stood out for me was this:

A Course in Miracles tells us that there is no such thing as a faithless person. Faith is an aspect of consciousness. We either have faith in fear or we have faith in love, faith in the power of the world or faith in the power of God.

God is the love within us.
~Marianne Williamson

What is Consciousness and Waking Up?

A few years ago, I turned the page on my Louise Hay desk calendar and found the following affirmation that changed my life:

The point of power is always in the present moment.

That statement woke me up to the present moment for the first time. I thought about all the time I had wasted feeling sad over things that happened in the past, and worrying about the future. That statement grounded me in the present like nothing ever has. Now when I start to go into frenzy, worry or feel sadness, I remember to be in the present moment and a deep peace comes over me.

How many of us are caught up in our thoughts of worry about what will happen, despair over what has happened and purposely distract ourselves from the present moment? We walk around in a state of unconsciousness, keeping busy and rushing though life. We avoid pain, boredom, sadness and other uncomfortable feelings. There are plenty of distractions from our feelings: smart phones, the internet, television, work, food, alcohol, drugs and getting involved in other people's drama.

♥ **Health Coach Wisdom:** When you decide you want to be more conscious, you can use distractions as a reminder to remain awake and be in the present moment. When the phone rings, or a loud commercial blasts, use it as an opportunity to wake up and connect with your soul. *Turn off the TV or shut off your ringer and be still.*

Learning about our personality, ego self, as opposed to our higher self has given me a pathway to guide my life. My life used to be about achieving; now it is about being my best self so that I can serve others. I aim to appreciate everything. I learned from Dr. Wayne Dyer, instead of thinking "What's in it for me? I now ask "How may I serve?" For me, being connected to a higher power also means being connected to everyone and everything on the planet. We create and send out energy. I want that energy to be loving, kind and a force for good. I trust that there is a force greater than me, guiding me to be my best self. In my experience Spirituality means believing in God, a higher power, which has helped me to alleviate my suffering and want to be a kinder more compassionate person. I have developed a technique that has helped me to rise above difficult situations. Instead of reacting quickly, I take a deep breath and ask "What what would my higher self say or do in this situation?"A deep sense of calm comes over me and I immediately get the correct answer and act with love and kindness. This works when I remember to connect instead of reacting without thinking.

There are two ways to live your life. One is as though nothing is
a miracle. The other is as though everything is a miracle.
~ Albert Einstein

You can choose to be greedy, controlling, interfering, judgmental, dark or fearful, or you can choose to be kind, sharing, open, allowing, accepting, and radiate light from a place of love. Unfortunately it is easy to become a slave to our habits. Becoming mindful and setting an intention to change something requires concentrated attention. Accepting that we have negative and positive feelings helps to make us whole. We don't need to fight against ourselves, we need to welcome our feelings and then choose how to feel and behave.

Years ago a good friend gave me the book, *The Four Agreements* by Don Miguel Ruiz, which had a profound impact on my personal growth. A former surgeon, Ruiz learned Toltec teachings from his family in Mexico. He combines ancient wisdom with modern insights. Realizing these tools would help people to be happier, he wrote *The Four Agreements* to help people transform their thoughts. Then he added a fifth agreement. He summarizes the Five Agreements this way:

The Five Agreements are tools to change your world. If you are impeccable with your words, if you don't take anything personally, if you don't make assumptions, if you always do your best, and if you are skeptical while listening, we won't have any more war in our head. There will be peace.

These are just concepts until we can put them into practice. My mentor, Erik Olesen, taught me that daily practice is a large part of spirituality. When we are aware of our intentions when things are difficult, when someone says something to offend us, or when we become angry, that is the time to work each one of the agreements as an exercise. Try it and watch your thoughts and actions shift. It is impossible to say hurtful things or to seek revenge when you are trying to be impeccable with your word or when you refuse to take what someone said personally. We can read hundreds of self-help books, but until we apply what we learn, we won't grow.

Once we begin down this spiritual path, we think it is going to be easy, and then when someone says something hurtful and we react badly, we think we have failed. We haven't failed, *it takes practice*. Erik also teaches "Progress, not perfection." Everything is a lesson. There is always another opportunity to "*not take it personally.*"

How Do We Keep From Taking Things Personally?

I was having a difference of opinion with my boss and I was getting upset. She asked me why I was taking the issue so personally, which upset me more. I didn't have an answer. It felt personal. I didn't realize it at the time, but this person was a gift, my spiritual teacher, helping me to change. I needed to grow and learn about my lower self, my ego, and my higher self. Later, she graciously took me to a group meeting for co-dependents, another turning point. I sought help from my therapist and studied this concept more. I learned why I felt so responsible and needed to be in control of everything. I learned that the need to control stems from fear. I found the concept of the higher self everywhere I turned. Many psychologists and spiritual teachers believe that we have a higher self, and what lives within is a place of peace, joy, compassion, appreciation, strength and love.

Susan Jeffers, who wrote *Feel the Fear and Do It Anyway*, said "The Higher Self is the spiritual part of who we are. Most of us live in the Lower Self, the place of struggle, lack, fear and pain." We all have incredible wisdom within us if we will get quiet and listen. Jeffers taught:

> If we do not consciously and consistently focus on the spiritual
> part of ourselves, we will never experience the kind of joy,
> satisfaction, safety and connectedness we are all seeking.
> ~ Susan Jeffers

"If you never rise above the level of the Lower Self, you will never feel free. If you transcend to the Higher Self, you will always feel free—despite what is happening in the outside world. You inner peace has nothing to do with the dramas of your life," adds

Jeffers. *Spirituality to me is living in the present moment, is being grateful for everything, good and the bad, and viewing "bad" as an opportunity to grow.*

♥ **Health Coach Wisdom:** It has been said that prayer is when we ask for something and meditation is when we listen for the answer.

How do you know when you are operating from your true self? You feel calm and at peace. You are clear and know deep down that you have the correct answer. You feel loving and non-judgmental.

There is a spiritual solution to every problem. ~ Dr. Wayne Dyer

When working with people as a Health and Wellness Coach I find it most difficult to convince people to be compassionate and forgiving with themselves. Many of us feel we have made poor choices that have led to problems and even shame. The longer we live, the more mistakes *we believe* we make. Unfortunately, our culture and some religions have taught us to feel guilt and shame, leading us to believe that we don't deserve to be happy and are beyond help. Self-forgiveness allows us to make mistakes, learn the lessons, repair the damage and move on. *If we can't see the goodness at our core, we won't be kind or compassionate with ourselves.*

Pema Chödrön is a beloved American Buddhist nun and author. Her teachings provide us with a strong vision of meeting each moment of our lives with greater wisdom, courage and compassion. She has a gift for explaining Buddhist teachings that resonate with our life experiences. She teaches that we already have everything we need, "there is no need for self-improvement." In her book *Pema Chödrön*, explains simply:

> All these trips that we lay on ourselves—the heavy-duty fearing that we're bad and hoping that we're good, the identities that we so dearly cling to, the rage, the jealousy and the addictions of all kinds—never touch our basic wealth. They are like clouds that temporarily block the sun. But all the time our warmth and brilliance are right here. This is who we really are. We are one blink of an eye away from being fully awake.

I have found peace in learning the teachings of the Buddhists philosophies which teach us that attachment causes suffering, that when we relax into our experiences and accept them things go more smoothly. I aim to practice the following Buddhist practice of the three vows:

1. Do no harm with our thoughts
2. Nurture our sense of compassion and dedicate our lives to ease the world's suffering
3. Embrace the world as it is

What is Enlightenment?

Charles A. Francis is the co-founder and director of the Mindfulness Meditation Institute. He has studied the practice of mindfulness with Zen Master Thich Nhat Hanh. For over 16 years, he has worked to help people find inner peace through mindfulness meditation. Charles is the author of *"Mindfulness in the Workplace: How organizations are using mindfulness to lower health care cost and increase productivity."* Charles Francis explains Enlightenment simply: **"I think Enlightenment is simply the evolution of human consciousness."**

According to Charles A. Francis, here are 12 of the qualities of an Enlightened Person:

1. **Happiness**: The enlightened person is happy and joyful.
2. **Peaceful and Serene**: Freedom from suffering comes from within, and not from material possessions.
3. **Loving, Kind, Compassionate**: Genuinely cares about other people, spiritually open to everyone.
4. **Not Self-Centered**: Realizing that all physical manifestations, humans, animals and plants depend on each other for their survival.
5. **Emotionally Stable**: The enlightened person is emotionally stable because he no longer has an ego that needs validation for its existence. He does not get angry because he is understanding and compassionate toward those who are not as far along the spiritual path.
6. **Patient and Understanding**: The enlightened person is patient and understanding because she appreciates how our ignorance creates our own suffering. She understands the challenge of becoming enlightened, so she doesn't condemn people for their missteps.
7. **Humble:** He doesn't need validation from others. Therefore, he has nothing to prove to anyone.
8. **Insightful and Open-Minded**: The enlightened person is able to see the world with great clarity, without attachment to preconceived ideas about people, places and things.
9. **Inner Strength:** The enlightened person has great inner strength. He has learned healthy ways of connecting with the sources of mindfulness energy-though healthy interactions with people and within. He no longer has a need for the power struggles that most of us engage in.

10. **Leadership**: The enlightened person is a leader. Having awakened to the point of understanding the nature of suffering, she realizes her duty to help other people find freedom from suffering. She leads by example, rather than control.

11. **Mindful of Health**: The enlightened person is mindful of his health-physical, mental and emotional. He knows that the mind, body and spirit must be in harmony in order to maintain his spiritual condition. He doesn't impair his mind with alcohol or illicit drugs.

12. **Committed to their Spiritual Practice**: The enlightened person never forgets how to achieve enlightenment. She is also aware that it takes continual effort to remain that way. It takes a great deal of mindfulness energy to help others along their path, so she's aware she needs to replenish her spiritual strength on a daily basis. Overall, the enlightened person is mindful of himself and the world around him. Furthermore, he is curious and willing to continue learning.

Happiness is a spiritual path. The more you learn about true happiness, the more you discover the truth of who you are, what is important, and what your life is for.
~ Dr. Robert Holden

In an article entitled *Mind Training for Today, in Shambala Sun Magazine* Zen teacher Norman Fischer sheds light on staying on your spiritual path:

> If your practice only works when things go well—if you turn away from it when things fall apart, if you don't know how to turn your difficulties into strength and wisdom—then your work probably won't be very effective. If, on the other hand, you are able to increase your forbearance and open your heart even more in the face of serious setbacks, you will have achieved the most prized of all spiritual accomplishments: the ability to continuously deepen your strength and love, no matter what happens.

When I entered into my health and wellness coach training, I was surprised to find a psychology based curriculum which included spirituality. We learned that beliefs about a higher purpose and meaning of the universe contribute to our well-being. When I discovered that our psychology-based training connects spirituality with wellness, I was convinced. *Spirituality is not a separate chapter in my book or a spoke on my wellness wheel; it is our center.*

I became fascinated with character strengths and virtues as these give us something *positive to aim for* rather than being consumed with *what's wrong with us*. In spirituality, words such as love, faith, joy, peace, awe and bliss are used to describe God and a feeling of being connected to our higher power. Other strengths we possess are awe, wonder and elevation, noticing and appreciating beauty and excellence. What is of key importance for well-being is gratitude.

> *My yoga teacher, Patricia Carpizo Kauffman shares many of her meditations and spiritual teachings with our class. One evening near the end of class, as we sat in a brief mediation, she shared with us a secret that she learned from her meditation teacher. This secret can make anyone happy in an instant. She told us that it opens the heart to grace and allows us to see every event as a blessing. It helps us to appreciate the earth, our air, water and things that we take for granted. She told us that this secret lifts us out of isolation and frees us from worry and that when we remember this one thing, our heart rests. I wondered what it was..."***Gratitude***" *she said quietly. I have never heard a word that has had a greater impact on me. Now when I start to get down or afraid I remember to be grateful and my mood shifts immediately.*

If you live in awareness, it is easy to see miracles everywhere.
~ Marianne Williamson

How do we Become Mindful?

How difficult do you find it to remember to be in the present moment? Thich Nhat Hanh, the highly respected Zen Buddhist monk, says to "Connect your mind with your body by breathing in, slowly with intention. Focus on your breath. Under the influence of awareness, you become more attentive, understanding, and loving, and your presence not only nourishes you and makes you lovelier, it enhances them as well. Our entire society can be changed by one person's peaceful presence."According to Thich Nhat Hanh, *The Heart Sutra* says that there is 'nothing to attain.' We meditate not to attain enlightenment, because enlightenment is already in us. We don't have to search anywhere."

Whenever we meditate, it changes our brain, and slows down our frantic thinking. We operate through our daily lives on automatic pilot, listening to the same old thoughts running through our heads. We get up every day and do the same things in the same ways. We tell ourselves that it is "hard" to change. Yet, when we practice mindfulness and meditation, focusing on our breath, focusing on each step, slowing down, right there—in the moment—this is where we gain the opportunity to change.

> *My mentor and therapist, Erik, encouraged me to meditate daily. At first, I spent only a few minutes here and there. It was not a habit. I have been a good student and developed all the healthy habits I have written about, but I had not given in to devote time to meditate. When I finally began to practice*

*meditating for fifteen or more minutes daily, I felt a shift and a deeper sense
of calm. It connects me to my higher self.*

When you begin to be still and learn to meditate, you will understand the difference between your higher awareness and your ego, the chatter voices in your head. This awareness is your power. You are not powerless over sugar, over your spending habits, over anything. You may not be aware of your power until you wake up to the present moment. Marianne Williamson points out in *A Return to Love*, "When we meditate, our brains literally emit different brain waves. We receive information at a deeper level of than we do during normal waking consciousness."

What are *your* spiritual practices? Praying, meditating, walking in nature, gardening, are some of the answers I received from interviewing people.

Choosing to be positive and having a grateful attitude is going
to determine how you are going to live your life.
~Joel Osteen

Positive Emotions and Spirituality

The positive emotions that create meaning are love, compassion, hope, awe, gratitude, forgiveness, trust and joy. These emotions are, according to Charles Darwin, the forces that help us to break out of our ego and self centeredness.

George E. Villant, M.D., is a psychoanalyst, a research psychiatrist, and professor at Harvard University directing Harvard's Study of Adult Development for thirty-five years. "Experiencing and giving love ignites the sense of our own efficacy as no belief in self-importance can. Attachment and compassion create positive satisfaction and the sense of fulfillment. The world's great religions–Buddhism, Hinduism, Christianity, Islam and Judaism– share two things in common: they are all based, in part, upon a commitment to unselfish love and have all endured for more than 1400 years," reports Dr. Villant. He explains that "The effect of positive emotion on the autonomic nervous system has much in common with the relaxation response to meditation that was popularized by a Harvard professor of medicine Herbert Benson. Indeed, positive emotion and spiritual experience cannot be disentangled."

The fight-or-flight response of negative emotion activates the sympathetic nervous system. In contrast, positive emotion activates the parasympathetic nervous system. Meditation brings positive emotions, such as joy, compassion, attachment, trust and forgiveness that reduce blood pressure, heart rate, and muscle tension.

Love goes very far beyond the physical person of the beloved. It finds
its deepest meaning in his spiritual being, his inner self.
~Viktor E. Frankl, *Man's Search for Meaning*

Our true nature *is* happiness, joy and well-being. It is encouraging to find that psychiatry is moving more toward the positive, and that spirituality and religion are more about the collective good than selfishness and greed. It is my belief that many people begin to feel disappointed and angry at themselves for the "mistakes" *they think* they have made. Some people feel "less than" for many reasons. Some people feel that they fail to live up to cultural norms. Our regrets start to eat away at us, and before too long, we may give up trying. We stay in a comfort zone of pretending to be all right or accepting misery. As time goes on, we settle for less than what we dreamed of. Here is the twist. We are not less than anyone else for not achieving a certain level of education, a certain title, marital status or for making mistakes—*we are good at our core. That is our true self.*

We learn and grow from our mistakes if we can forgive ourselves and others. The irony is that is if people trusted and believed that we are good—that we are not *our mistakes*, we would not continue making poor choices, making life difficult for ourselves and those around us. When we don't believe in ourselves, we don't value taking care of our physical bodies and our minds. *Many lost people continue on a dark path unless they realize they are to be valued as they are.*

What I have found to be the most compelling, and most powerful force to help people turn their life around, is taking hold of spirituality in whatever form that speaks to them. Unfortunately, what often happens is that Spirituality, the very thing that brings most people great comfort, is often misunderstood and can prevent some people from being open to a higher power.

Man can no longer live for himself alone. We realize that all life is valuable,
and that we are united to this life. From this knowledge comes our
spiritual relationship to the universe. ~Albert Schweitzer, scientist

How Can We Be Compassionate With Ourselves?

I haven't yet found the answer to why we are so hard on ourselves, but I have found ways that we can practice being kinder and more compassionate with our self- talk and our actions. First we have to notice what we are saying to ourselves, and how we are neglecting our self-care. When we make a mistake, instead of saying "Oh, you did it again, "we could say to our self, "you'll do better next time."

Jack Kornfield, Buddhist teacher and author, teaches that in our culture, people find it difficult to direct loving-kindness to themselves. So rather than start loving-kindness practice with ourselves, he suggests it more helpful to start with those we most naturally love and care about. "We open our heart in the most natural way, and then direct our loving-kindness little by little to areas where it's more difficult. Think of someone you care about and love a lot. Then let natural phrases of good wishes for them come into your mind and heart," such as:

- ♥ May you be safe and protected
- ♥ May you be healthy and strong
- ♥ May you be truly happy.

Kornfield says to extend this kindness to another person you care about, then another, until you turn them toward yourself. "May I be safe and protected. May I be healthy and strong. May I be truly happy."

♥ **Health Coach Wisdom:** If you practice loving-kindness meditation for a few minutes per day, you will begin to calm anxious, worried, fearful or angry thoughts, and begin to develop new patterns of thinking and being.

I resisted listening to God most of my life and I remained in a state of confusion for years until I began to feel helpless. I searched to find something to make me strong. I wondered about God, but it wasn't until some of my relationships became strained and I couldn't stand the pain anymore that I knew I needed help. I turned to counseling, group meetings and self-help books. The ones that made the biggest impact were spiritual in nature. Many of our greatest leaders and teachers throughout history have been spiritual. Some of the finest minds of all time believe in a power greater than ourselves, that we are all connected in this vast universe and that love and compassion dissolve problems and bring peace. I soaked up spiritual ideas that brought me comfort. In addition to spiritual teachers, I read books by people whose lives had been transformed from suffering their own mental torments, depression and addictions to healing through spiritual teachings. And most importantly, I stayed connected to group support and my therapist and mentor, Erik Olesen. I didn't realize it at the time, but he shared with me a simple, yet powerful relaxation technique that was the beginning of my meditation practice. He encouraged me to think about and feel the feeling of the following words for ten seconds each: Gratitude, Peace, Love and Joy. Try it for yourself. It works to evoke these feelings immediately.

My hope is that people will begin to focus on religion and spirituality as a way to bring people together instead of driving us apart. The Dalai Lama said in 1985:

The world's religions can contribute to world peace if there is peace and growing harmony between different faiths. It would be tragic if inter-religious rivalry and conflict undermines world peace in the twenty-first century. I have always encouraged and supported efforts towards better understanding among different faiths. It is my firm belief that this better understanding will enhance the ability of different faiths to make positive contributions to world peace.

Alan Cohen in his book, *The Dragon Doesn't Live Here Anymore* reminded us what Jesus taught, "Love thy neighbor as thy self," and "Do unto others as you would have them do unto you." "He taught this because thy neighbor is thy self, and when we do unto others, we are doing unto yourself, "writes Cohen. As a spiritual teacher who has spent most of his life beautifully explaining religion and spirituality, I find myself most comforted by Alan Cohen's philosophies on life. Here is some gentle wisdom from him that may help heal us:

"As *we come to understand the implications of transference of our thoughts and feelings, we can use the principles to our advantage.* Until we do, we may feel like a leaf in the wind, at the mercy of the rampant energies of those around us. There are three ways in which we can capitalize on our understanding of how thoughts work:

1. Seek to be in the presence of positive people who share your ideals; place yourself in environments that support your spiritual growth.
2. Keep your clear, calm center when you are in the midst of negative thoughts and feelings; do not compromise your awareness of God's Perfect Presence.
3. Be a generator of positive and loving thoughts and feeling, so that you will enhance, and not detract from the experiences of those around you."

There can be no spirituality without loving-kindness.
~Dan Millman

In each moment we can choose to think and speak from the thoughts running through our personality, our ego mind or we can choose to feel with our heart and speak from our spiritual center. Our relationships, our health and our lives improve when we shift from our lower selves to our higher selves. This takes practice—*the practice we choose in each moment is what creates our life.* How is it possible to make this shift? We shift when we drop down into our hearts. Author Dan Millman offers guidance in his book, *Everyday Enlightenment:*

> Your heart is not just a muscle in your chest; it is also the mystical center of love. You can love as, from, and with your whole body and being, but every culture I've visited associates love with the heart. That muscle, quietly beating, pumping life through your body, is the center of love...It is known in numerous ancient spiritual and mystical traditions that we first connect with and experience the love and inspiration of our higher selves at the heart center.

As you have progressed through *Health Coach Wisdom,* hopefully you have begun to choose more positive thoughts, choose more nutritious foods, choose to move more throughout your day, choose to improve your relationships and choose to be more joyful—*to be more aware.* Spirituality means being fully aware, being present in the moment and for me means connecting with my higher power, creating a reverence for life and an appreciation for everything. Bringing spirituality into your life may be the key to making better choices out of love for yourself. I close with two affirmations, the first is from Louise Hay, and the second from me, was inspired by Alan Cohen.

My heart is the center of my power. I create easily and effortlessly when
I let my thoughts come from the loving space of my own heart.

~

Please help me to think and act
from my higher self
in each moment today.

Action Steps

Name three daily spiritual practices to help you connect with
your higher self, and then commit to doing them:

1. _____
2. _____
3. _____

What you choose to think, see and do in each moment is your spiritual message.
~Jeni Stepanek, PhD, *Mattie Stepanek's Mother*

Books and Resources

The Answer is Simple, Love Yourself, Live Your Spirit by Sonia Choquette, Hay House, 2009.

A Return To Love by Marianne Williamson, Harper Collins, 1992.

Holy Shift! 365 Daily Meditations from A Course in Miracles by Robert Holden, PHD, Hay House Inc. 2014.

The Abundance of Grace by Ingrid Goff-Maidoff, 2007, www.tendingjoy.com.

Everyday Enlightenment-The Twelve Gateways to Personal Growth, by Dan Millman, Warner Books, Inc. 1998.

The Purpose Driven Life by Rick Warren, Zondervan 2002.

A Deep Breath of Life~ Daily Inspiration for Heart-Centered Living by Alan Cohen, Hay House Inc. 1996.

The Seven Spiritual Laws of Success ~ A Practical Guide to the fulfillment of your dreams by Deepak Chopra, Amber-Allen Publishing and New World Library, 1994.

Mastering the Winds of Change: Peak Performers Reveal How to Stay on Top in Times of Turmoil by Erik Olesen, Rawson Associates, Macmillan Publishing. 1993.

The Shadow Effect by Deepak Chopra, Debbie Ford and Marianne Williamson. Audio book, e-book, and print. www.harperaudio.com, www.shadoweffect.com.

www.joelosteen.com: books, podcasts, weekly inspirational messages and more.

Chapter 7

Find Peace with Your Sense of Purpose

> The whole point of being alive is to evolve into the
> complete person you were intended to be.
> ~ Oprah Winfrey

We all need a purpose. We need to feel a sense of belonging, to feel needed, and to make a contribution. We all belong in this world, yet some of us feel isolated, and we do this to ourselves. If you are alive, *you belong* and you can connect with others as soon as you begin to value yourself. You do not have to do anything *to have* value. If you have made mistakes, learn from them and appreciate the opportunity to begin again. See how you can help someone else. Reaching out to others, either by helping them or asking for help provides meaning and connection in your life.

Embracing spirituality is healing to the mind, body and spirit. This brings us to our next step—our sense of purpose. Each step to wellness is no less important than another, and as explained in Maslow's Hierarchy of Needs, you won't feel like thinking about your purpose in life if you aren't taking care of your basic needs. If you have been *working* this book, and not just reading it, hopefully, you have made some changes. You may feel better about yourself and have the desire to think about your purpose, which will bring more meaning to your life. This, in turn, will give you the motivation to continue taking good care of your physical and mental health. *Life is short and there is little time to be discontented. Bringing your awareness to what gives your life purpose will point you in a meaningful direction.*

People who's happiness stems from being good to others and feeling a deep sense of purpose have less active inflammatory genes and more active antiviral ones, which combine for a stronger immune system, according to research from The University of California, Los Angeles. The Dalai Lama says, "Our prime purpose in this life is to help others. And if you can't help them, at least don't hurt them."

> For the world is in a bad state, but everything will become
> still worse unless each of us does his best.
> ~Viktor E. Frankl, *Man's Search for Meaning*

Having a sense of purpose is one of the pillars of our health, yet according to the Center for Disease Control, about 4 out of 10 Americans have not discovered a satisfying life purpose. Research has shown that having purpose and meaning in life increases overall well-being and life satisfaction, improves mental and physical health, enhances resiliency, enhances self-esteem, and decreases the chances of depression.

Having a sense of purpose does not have to be difficult. In the last chapter, we learned that being connected to something bigger than ourselves helps us to heal. The Mayo Clinic reports, "Whatever form your spirituality takes—religious observance, prayer, meditation, belief in a higher power—*connecting to what's meaningful and feeling part of a greater whole can bring inner peace and a sense of purpose.*

> To be a loving presence is the greatest contribution you
> make in any situation you find yourself in.
> ~ Dr. Robert Holden

If you don't yet know your purpose, don't be discouraged. *I believe we have many purposes throughout our lives.* If you have children, your purpose is raising them well. If you have aging parents, your purpose at this time in your life may be caring for them. If you have a job, your purpose is doing it the best you can while uplifting those around you. If what you are doing now doesn't feel like "enough", you can express your creativity, paint, write, garden, volunteer with a worthy cause or do whatever gives you satisfaction. I have a client in her eighties who is an accomplished artist and author who *is still working.* She says, *"Everyone has something to contribute. We need to give back. I am grateful and say thank you every day."*

At various stages in our lives we have different purposes. Balancing your life by creating health and harmony within is one of your most important purposes. When you are ready, when your health is good, you can begin to discover the purpose that calls to you. Don't be hard on yourself. Take your time and enjoy the journey. Our purpose is to align our personalities with our higher selves—to be more loving, kind, joyous and compassionate. In any moment, ask, "What would my higher self do now?" "What kind of person do I want to be and what kind of contribution will I make while on this earth?" At any moment, you can express the highest within yourself.

> Connection is what brings purpose and meaning to our lives.
> ~ Brene Brown

The Secret to Living is Giving.
~ Tony Robbins

Viktor Frankl was a psychiatrist who survived The Holocaust, in spite of losing his pregnant wife, parents and most of his family in a Nazi concentration camp. He survived unimaginable horrors for three years and when he was freed in 1946, he wrote the book, *Man's Search for Meaning*. Frankl concluded that the difference between those who had lived and those who had died came down to one thing: Meaning. As he saw in the camps, those who found meaning even in the most horrendous circumstances were far more resilient to suffering than those who did not. "Everything can be taken from a man but one thing," Frankl wrote, "the last of the human freedoms—to choose one's attitude in any given set of circumstances, to choose one's own way." Frankl helped inmates in the camps realize there was still something they needed to survive for. For Frankl, it was to live to write the story of what happened. He ultimately developed logotherapy, a contribution to clinical psychology, *which helps people overcome depression and achieve well-being by finding their unique meaning in life.*

Writer Emily Esfahani, in an article in The Atlantic about Frankl, explained why meaningfulness matters more than happiness: "*A man who becomes conscious of the responsibility he bears toward a human being who affectionately waits for him, or to an unfinished work, will never be able to throw away his life. He knows the 'why' for his existence, and will be able to bear any 'how'.*"

As long as you are breathing, it is never too late to do some good.
~ Maya Angelou

Norman Fischer is a Zen teacher and founder of the Everyday Zen Foundation. In his book, Training in Compassion, he talks about how we are dependent on others to make our clothes, build our homes and grow our food. The Buddhists teach that there is no such thing as an isolated individual. We are what we are *because of other people*. He advises how to "be grateful to everyone." In an article from Shambala Sun Magazine, "Life is Tough", Fischer writes:

> It is to cultivate every day this sense of gratitude, the happiest of all attitudes. Unhappiness and gratitude simply cannot exist in the same moment. If you feel grateful, you are a happy person. If you feel grateful that you are alive at all, that you can think, that you can feel, that you can stand, sit, walk talk—if you feel grateful, you are happy and maximize your chances for well-being and for sharing happiness with others.

> When you are feeling helpless, help someone else.
> See the miracle that is this life.
> ~ Marie Forleo, business coach

Do you want to skyrocket past feeling down, helpless or like a victim? Do you want to find greater meaning and purpose in your life? Find one thing you can do each day to make someone's day brighter. If you are taking care of other people, make sure you are not acting out of guilt or obligation. Then, do something nurturing for yourself.

> *One lesson I have learned from my mentor, Erik Olesen, is how to balance how we help others. When he shared with me that it is not always helpful to do something for others when they are capable of doing it themselves, I knew I found the answer to the question I was seeking. I enjoy doing things for other people and making them happy. But I was crossing boundary lines. Often, I drain my own energy and push myself taking care of others when I need some self-care, or I do things that I'm not asked to do. I used to cross lines thinking I was being helpful, when I was really being annoying. Now I am more aware. So how do you know the difference? Get quiet, and ask your heart, "Will this be helpful? Will this make someone's day? Will it ease another's loneliness or make their life easier? Or do I need to let them handle things their own way?"*

> Decide upon your major definite purpose in life
> and then organize all your activities around it.
> ~ Brian Tracy

♥ **Health Coach Wisdom:** Finding the balance between doing for others and doing for ourselves is essential to our health and well-being.

Pema Chödrön explains how in *Living Beautifully,* "Compassion is not a matter of pity or the strong helping the weak; it's a relationship between equals, one of mutual support… we come to realize that other people's welfare is just as important as our own. In helping them, we help ourselves. In helping ourselves, we help the world."

Perhaps one of the world's greatest authorities on Life Purpose is Deepak Chopra, a leader in the fields of holistic health and human potential. In his book, *The Seven Spiritual Law of Success,* he writes:

Everyone has a purpose in life...a unique gift of special talent to give to others. And when we blend this unique talent with service to others, we experience the ecstasy and exultation of our own spirit, which is the ultimate goal of all goals.

Deepak teaches that the seventh spiritual law of success is the Law of Dharma, a Sanskrit word that means "purpose in life." He says that we need to have three commitments if we want to make maximum use of the Law of Dharma:

1. I am going to seek my higher self, which is beyond my ego, through my spiritual practice.
2. I am going to discover my unique talents. (*This is when I am in a state of bliss.*)
3. I am going to ask myself how I am best suited to serve humanity.

Love is our ultimate reality and our purpose on earth. To be consciously aware of it, to experience love in ourselves and others, is the meaning of life.
~ Marianne Williamson

In his book, *The Life You Were Born to Live ~A Guide to Finding Your Life Purpose,* author Dan Millman, lays out a roadmap to help people find new meaning, purpose and direction for our path. An important concept he explains is the Law of Choices:

The most basic choice we have in life is whether to expand or contract, whether to bring our creative and expressive energies out into the world in positive or negative ways. No matter what our circumstances, we have the power to choose our directions.

Be a good example of how to live a wonderful life.
~Elizabeth Gilbert, author of *Eat, Pray, Love*

It takes courage to step out of your comfort zone and make changes. It is easier, yet still painful, to sit back and think that your dreams are out of reach. Those who live their dreams and purpose, people like Oprah Winfrey, Anthony Robbins, Dr. Wayne Dyer, Elizabeth Gilbert, Michael Jordan, and Taylor Swift all had a calling and acted on it—and they all serve others in their own way. It requires work, discipline and often disappointment, but those who have a purpose prevail. I've heard it said that "If you do what you love, you won't work a day in your life." We may not think we have super human talent like those mentioned above so we may not try. Dan Millman offers some guidance and inspiration for trying:

Discipline is the surest means to greater freedom and independence; it provides the focus to achieve the skill level and depth of knowledge that translates into more options in life. What we all need is a clear purpose—a meaningful goal or mission that connects us with other human beings.

♥ **Health Coach Wisdom:** Becoming aware and living joyfully in the present moment gives you courage to share your gifts and talents.

Some people regard discipline as a chore.
For me, it is a kind of order that sets me free to fly.
~Julie Andrews

Eckhart Tolle in his book, *A New Earth, Awakening to Your Life's Purpose,* explains the difference between your *inner purpose and your outer purpose:*

As soon as you rise above mere survival, the question of meaning and purpose becomes of paramount importance in your life...There is no substitute for finding true purpose. But the true or primary purpose of your life cannot be found on the outer level. It does not concern what you do but what you are—that is to say, your state of consciousness...Your life has an inner purpose and an outer purpose. Inner purpose concerns being and is primary. Outer purpose concerns doing and is secondary. Your inner purpose is to awaken. It is as simple as that.

Awakening is a shift in consciousness in which thinking and awareness separate...Instead of being lost in your thinking, when you are awake you recognize yourself as the awareness behind it...The initiation of the awakening process is an act of grace.

Jack Canfield, author of *The Success Principals,* teaches us how to discover your purpose. In this powerful book, Jack Canfield helps us to clarify the "why" behind what we do. He says, "Without purpose as the compass to guide you, your goals and action plans may not ultimately fulfill you." When you are working toward something important, and are in alignment with your purpose, you want to take care of your mind and body without hesitation.

Jack Canfield's life purpose exercise from *The Success Principals helped me to clarify mine*:

1. List two of your unique personal qualities, such as *creativity* and *enthusiasm.*
2. List one or two ways you enjoy expressing those qualities when interacting with others, such as *to support* and *to inspire.*
3. Assume the world is perfect right now. What does this world look like? How is everyone interacting with everyone else? What does it feel like? Write your answer as a statement, in the present tense, describing the ultimate condition, the perfect world as you see it and feel it. *Remember, a perfect world is a fun place to be.*
4. Combine the three prior subdivisions into a single statement.

Here is an example of my life purpose: My purpose is to use my <u>compassion</u> and <u>vision</u> to <u>inspire</u> and <u>support</u> others in getting clear on how to create a healthy and harmonious lifestyle.

Now create your own life purpose! Write it here:

_____

_____

_____

_____.

I also believe my purpose is to communicate ideas and information in a simple way to help people live better lives. I have researched the definition of PURPOSE from leading authorities. Here are some inspirational quotes to guide you in finding your purpose:

It is not what we get, but who we become, what we contribute that gives meaning to our lives. Life is a gift and it offers us the privilege, opportunity and responsibility to give something back by becoming something more. ~ Anthony Robbins

Choosing to be positive and having a grateful attitude is going to determine how you are going to live your life. ~ Joel Osteen

The evolution of your consciousness is why you are here.
It's your purpose. ~ Cheryl Richardson

The only person you are destined to become is the person you decide to be.
~ Ralph Waldo Emerson

The purpose of life is joy.
~Louise Hay

167

It is what we decide to be—who we are. It's about what we bring to what we do. What we bring to every situation. We give everything purpose and meaning. Our purpose is to be our best self.
~ Carolyn Myss

The meaning of life is to find your gift.
The purpose of life is to give it away.
~ Brian Tracy

When you perceive your own light, you become complete, fulfilled, and free.
~ Patricia Kauffman, *Padma and the Blue Castle*

When you make love your purpose
You are fulfilling your destiny.
~ Dr. Robert Holden

Action Steps: To find meaning and purpose in your life, contemplate the following questions and write the answers when you are ready.

If I didn't have to make a living, what would I do for work or to volunteer? _____
_____.

What do I love to do? What are my gifts and talents? _____
_____.

What can I do to ease the suffering of others? To help protect our planet?_____
_____.

How can I best serve others? How can I make a difference in the world? _____
_____.

What did I love to do as a child or young person? What brings me joy? _____
_____.

What are the reoccurring themes and patterns in my life? _____
_____.

How can I use the sorrows and lessons of my life to benefit others? _____
_____.

Follow your passion. It will lead you to your purpose.
~ Oprah Winfrey

In thinking about ways to fulfill your purpose, you can turn to those in need of attention and care. What speaks to your heart? Think about the people who need your help such as injured veterans, helpless children, the elderly or abused animals. *Choose your own cause or review the following list of organizations that are of service to people, children, animals and our environment. They are able to do good work because of people like you who help with donations of money or time.*

The ASPCA, www.aspca.org and **The Humane Society of the United States**, www.humanesociety.org are in constant battles to end animal neglect, cruelty and abuse. Your donation helps provide security and safety for abused and neglected animals. You can volunteer, make a donation or adopt a pet.

St. Jude Children's Research Hospital: www.st.jude.org. St. Jude provides lifesaving care for children with cancer and is working to drive the overall survival rate for childhood cancer to 90 percent in the next decade.

Habitat for Humanity www.habitat.org is a nonprofit organization that seeks to eliminate poverty housing and homelessness from the world. They invite people of all backgrounds, races and religions to build houses together in partnership with families in need. For more information or to volunteer your time or donate visit their website.

Help Children in Foster Care: There are several hundred thousand children in foster care in the United States who have been physically or sexually abused and neglected. There are many ways to make a difference in a child's life other than being a foster parent. Check with your local Foster Care Agency. Here are ways you can help:

- Provide emergency care for a short time, anywhere from 24 hours to 30 days.
- Become a CASA-Court Appointed Special Advocate. CASA workers are volunteers (angels) that work with the court and the foster homes to see that children are not lost in the system. They are the voice for the child.
- Be a Big Brother or Sister. You can spend about 3-4 hours a week with a child and make a difference. Taking time for a child is an amazing gift.
- Volunteer at a children's home. Children are first taken there when they are first removed from a neglectful or abusive situation.
- Donate clothes, toys, shoes, school supplies, toiletries and needed items in good condition. *Many children leave the children's home with what little belongings they have in a trash bag.* You can collect tote bags for these children and teens.

World Concern: www.worldconcern.org. Your donation of 44 cents provides de-worming medicine for poverty stricken children. You can restore a child living in extremely poor conditions to health. World Concern also provides clean water, sanitation and hygiene training to some of the driest places in the world and offers services to protect children from trafficking, works to stop the spread of Ebola.

Charity Water: www.charitywater.org. Water affects everything from health to poverty. A child under five dies every minute as a result of contaminated water. Charity water helps by providing clean water to save lives around the world.

No Kid Hungry: Share Our Strength: www.nokidhungry.org. Help eliminate childhood hunger in America. One in five kids struggles with hunger in America.

Anthony Robbins Foundation: www.anthonyrobbinsfoundation.org provides food, clothing and hope to those in need. Teaming with www.feedingamerica.org, Tony Robbins is providing 50 million meals this year, doing his part to end hunger. *17 million children in America go to bed hungry each night.*

The American Heart Association. www.heart.org. Resources for the prevention of heart disease. Help with stress management, nutrition, workplace wellness and more.

> Did you know that choosing to follow the guidance of your Higher Self gives you more freedom than you ever imagined was possible? It allows you to live an authentic, loving, fearless life. Nothing gives you more power than that. Just decide you want your Higher Self to run your life, and say so in no uncertain terms. It's the most direct way to realize all your dreams.
> ~ Sonia Choquette, author and spiritual teacher

Books and Resources:

The Life You Were Born to Live- A Guide To Finding Your Life Purpose by Dan Millman, New World Library, 1993, www.peacefulwarrior.com.

A New Earth~Awakening to Your Life's Purpose by Eckhart Tolle, Plume Group, 2006.

The Success Principles, How to Get from Where You Are to Where You Want to Be, by Jack Canfield, Harper Collins Publishers, 2005.

Padma and the Blue Castle by Patricia Carpizo Kauffman, Balboa Press, 2012.

Just who will you be? by Maria Shriver,, Hyperion Books, 2008.

Tune in–Let Your Intuition Guide You To Fulfillment and Flow by Sonia Choquette, Hay House, Inc., 2011.

Finding Your Passion by Cheryl Richardson, (audio program), Hay House Inc., 2004.

Chapter 8

Sleeping Well and Other Wellness Strategies

First, say to yourself
What you would be;
Then do what you have to do.
~ Epictetus

Being well takes self awareness, focus, and consistent action. Wellness is built on healthy habits. So if we know what to do, so why don't we do it? I have found that most people don't put their health first. We often put everything else ahead of taking care of ourselves. Why? We forget, we are busy, we don't have systems for maintaining our health and we talk ourselves out of doing things that hurt us because we are not in enough pain or discomfort to make changes. *The biggest obstacle is not facing what is bothering us.* We use distractions such as food, alcohol, caffeine, drugs, spending money, gambling, technology, and drama to avoid doing what we know is best for us.

Creating systems and making a daily plan will assure that you develop and maintain habits that help you to thrive. Below is a sample daily health schedule. Write your own and post it where you will see it as a reminder to take care of yourself.

<u>Sample Daily Health Schedule</u>

- ♥ Drink a glass of water with lemon first thing in the morning
- ♥ Fill my 64 ounce water jug to drink throughout the day
- ♥ Read something uplifting, meditate or enjoy some quiet time
- ♥ Eat a healthy breakfast, prepare lunch to take to work, review dinner plan
- ♥ Walk on breaks at work, move at least 5 out of 60 minutes each hour
- ♥ Eat a healthy lunch, take my vitamins, eat a nutritious afternoon snack
- ♥ Do my 30-60 minutes of walking or exercise as planned on my calendar
- ♥ Plan my to-do list for the next day

- ♥ Go to bed by 10 pm. Limit computer and screen time after 8 pm.
- ♥ Count the people and things I am grateful for as I drift off to sleep

Action is the antidote to despair.
~ Joan Baez

It is very common for people to wait until they have a heart attack, a stroke, a diagnosis of type 2 diabetes or receive bad news from the dentist until they are motivated enough to make lasting change—*if they survive the event.* The answer to developing healthy habits is to 1) put your awareness on healthy habits 2) believe you can develop them, and 3) then decide you will do what it takes. It becomes easy to fit better habits into your lifestyle if you know what your reasons are for changing. If you remember why you are making the change, you will be more empowered to act consistently toward your goal of preventing illness and disaster from striking you.

Getting Good Sleep-*Why Does it Matter?*

Why does it matter if we brush and floss our teeth? Why does it matter if we stay up late and watch a movie? You can talk yourself out of doing almost anything that is good for you by saying to yourself, "What does it matter?" In fact, most people put off doing what they need to, until there is a problem. One area that most people agree upon is wishing for a better night's sleep.

Why does it matter if you get enough sleep? Just as with eating well and getting exercise, getting enough sleep is a critical factor in preventing illness, strengthening our immune system and affecting how we feel. Unfortunately, for many of us, a complete night of rest seems impossible. Yet there are many things you can do to sleep better. The quality of your sleep depends on the choices you make throughout your day. *You have the ability to improve your sleep patterns without taking medication!*

Sleeping well is not only a key to good health, but also to your weight. The better quality your sleep is, the more balanced your hormones are, causing you to be more active and eat less. In recent years there have been a number of studies suggesting that insufficient sleep increases the risk of gaining weight, developing diabetes and even getting some cancers. Research has shown that sleep deprivation can have a significant impact on your ability to lose weight. The reasons for this are two hormones, leptin and ghrelin. Lack of sleep results in lower levels of the appetite-suppressing leptin and higher levels of the appetite-boosting ghrelin.

Researchers from German Universities Tubingen, Lubeck and Uppsala University in Sweden found that when we are sleep deprived we move around less and eat more. In fact, *the shorter amount of time volunteers in the study slept, the hungrier they were!* When we sleep less, we also have more opportunities to snack out of boredom. Also, when we're tired we have less will to fight cravings and mindless eating.

Now that you know more reasons to get enough sleep, you may be even more worried about not sleeping well. There is no need to panic. The following strategies can help you get a restful night's sleep if you follow them. A key step to sleeping well is to learn how to shut off your thoughts and stop worrying!

♥ **Health Coach Wisdom:** The key to a good night's sleep is to recognize that worrying is useless. Do what you can during the day to take care of yourself, your family, your finances, your job and then at night—let it all go. When those thoughts creep in, shut them down. Tell yourself there is nothing you can do in the middle of the night, and if you sleep well, you will make better decisions in the daytime. *Instead of counting sheep, count all the things you are grateful for.*

What Don't You Sleep Well?

Once you have read through the strategies for sleeping well, sit quietly and write down what keeps you up at night. We can control our thoughts and seek help when we need to. Research shows that people who sleep too little over many nights don't perform as well on complex mental tasks as do people who get closer to seven hours of sleep each night. Studies among adults also show that *getting less or much more* than *seven to eight hours of sleep* a night is associated with a higher mortality rate. School age children need *nine to eleven hours of sleep.* Lack of sleep is a real problem for kids and teens who stay up late using their computers and phones, yet must wake up early for school. *Once I have worked with clients for a short time, their sleep improves by utilizing a few of the following strategies:*

A Plan to Help You Sleep 7-8 Hours Each Night
Tips for helping you build better sleep habits:

- ♥ **Believe and affirm**: You have within you the power to create a good night's sleep and the ability to wake up feeling refreshed and well rested.
- ♥ **Goal**: Set a goal to get consistent, peaceful sleep, to fall asleep easily and go back to sleep quickly if woken in the night. Overcome the fear of not sleeping.

- ♥ **Change the pattern**: Many people have trouble falling asleep, staying asleep, tuning out the day's problems and worrying about the future. You can create new sleeping habits by going to bed and waking at the same time each day.
- ♥ **Understand the causes of poor sleep.** These include working at the computer within two hours of bedtime, listening to the news or upsetting shows before retiring, overeating, excessive alcohol, and unresolved worry.

Finish each day and be done with it…You have done what you could; some blunders and absurdities no doubt crept in; forget them as soon as you can. Tomorrow is a new day; you shall begin it well and serenely.
~ Ralph Waldo Emerson

Sleep Solution Strategies: Sweet Dreams

- ♥ Do something relaxing before bed time. Using relaxation techniques such as breathing and meditation can help you to do away with nagging thoughts. Listen to soft music, journal or read.
- ♥ Organize before you go to bed and make a "Things I Want to Do" list for the next day to relieve your mind. *If you phrase it in the positive and put it on paper you empower yourself to do the things you choose to do.*
- ♥ Don't go to bed mad.
- ♥ Praise yourself for the things you did right today, rather than thinking about the things you didn't do.
- ♥ Think of things you are grateful for as you drift off to sleep. *This works!*
- ♥ Put sleep on your priority list! *What you do through the day affects your sleep.*
- ♥ Create a peaceful sanctuary in your bedroom by rearranging your furniture and un-cluttering your bedroom. Your bedroom should be clean, clutter and dust free with no distractions. No TV, computer or desk if possible. If you are short on space, place a divider or screen around your work area to block your office work.
- ♥ Paint your bedroom soothing colors and hang calming and beautiful artwork.

Your bedroom should be a place for rest, a safe haven for you.

Your Sleeping Environment
Essentials for good sleep

- ♥ A room temperature of 62-68 degrees is best.
- ♥ Good ventilation is important- crack a window or use a fan or air filter.

- ♥ Invest in a quality mattress and pillows. Keep linens freshly washed.
- ♥ Turn off TVs, computers or phones—move them away from you.
- ♥ Create a bedtime routine. This is especially important for children! **Turn down lights in your home two hours before bedtime to help your natural melatonin start inducing sleep.** Block lights from electronics that can keep you awake.
- ♥ Keeping your bedroom dark promotes good sleep.
- ♥ Try using a sleep mask and/or ear plugs in noisy environments.
- ♥ Get plenty of fresh air and sunshine during the day to establish your circadian rhythms to wake your brain up. *This is nature's best health secret.*

Your Physical Strategies
Prerequisites for Good Sleep

- ♥ Cut out caffeine after noon or at least 8 hours before your bedtime.
- ♥ Eat dinner early and keep bedtime snacks light, no greasy or spicy foods. What you eat can disrupt your sleep by creating heartburn or making you sick.
- ♥ Watch out for alcohol and tobacco- alcohol may help you fall asleep, *but will wake you up and prevent you from going back to sleep. Tobacco will keep you up.*
- ♥ Watch out for medications- some can cause sleep*less*ness. Read labels.
- ♥ Establish good sleep patterns. Go to sleep at the same time each night and wake up 7-8 hours later. Children and teenagers need 9-11 hours of sleep.
- ♥ Exercise and physical activity calms you and helps you sleep more soundly.

♥ **Health Coach Wisdom:** Eat nutritious foods that help you sleep and strengthen your immune system. Sleep deprivation dampens the production of the antibodies needed to fight infection; while getting adequate sleep boosts your mood and gives you more energy to exercise, both of which can help strengthen your immunity.

Wellness Strategies
Health Maintenance ~ Self Care Check List

Visiting your doctor can empower you with knowledge about your health numbers and inspire you to make better choices. With that in mind, let's look at some other areas that are essential to building your healthy life. When it comes to your self-care, you may want to add these items to your check list:

- ✓ Annual Physical Check ups
- ✓ Dental Care and Exams and Eye Care (Ophthalmologist or Optometrist)
- ✓ Dermatologist (to check for skin cancers)
- ✓ Foot Care (Podiatrist) or wear shoes that support your feet and activity

---

♥ **Health Coach Wisdom:** Keep a Health Maintenance Checklist of everything you need to keep your body in tip top shape and follow through. *If you can do it for your car, then you can do it for your mind and body!*

How Heart Health is Connected to Your Teeth

One of the people I look most forward to seeing is my dentist, Dr. Roger Haddad. He is a gentle, caring and knowledgeable dentist who explains *the why* behind taking good care of your teeth and gums. Dr. Haddad shares why he feels proper dental hygiene is important:

> Are you avoiding the dentist? You might want to change your mind. Recent studies have shown that people with gum disease or periodontal disease are twice as likely to also have Coronary Artery Disease. The same inflammation that causes gum disease also causes inflammation in other parts of your body including your heart, lungs and joints. Therefore, keep your mouth healthy—see your dentist today!
>
> ~Dr. Roger Haddad, MS, DDS

When my family and I first started going to Dr. Haddad many years ago, he and his staff expertly explained the benefits of flossing carefully, using electric toothbrushes, water picks and taking excellent care our teeth and gums. I listened because of the heart disease and periodontal disease in my family history. Dr. Haddad says that my taking good care of my teeth and gums is paying off. And my whole family has benefited from good oral hygiene practice. Many people don't listen when it comes to getting regular dental check-ups and cleanings. If you want to avoid the high cost of neglecting dental care, both with your wallet and your heart health, make going to the dentist part of your healthy habit routine.

♥ **Health Coach Wisdom:** Researchers believe that inflammation from gum disease allows bacteria to enter your mouths blood vessels, travel into the coronary artery vessels, and narrow their passages. This reduces blood flow, which hurts the heart. Keep your mouth healthy. Make it a habit to brush 2-3 times per day and floss daily.

Reasons to Change Unhealthy Habits

Smoking and Chewing Tobacco: *According to the U.S. Department of Health and Human Services,* smoking is the leading preventable cause of death in the United States. Cigarette smoking causes more than 480,000 deaths each year in the U.S. If you smoke, get the help you need to quit. Here are a few more reasons to stop:

- Smoking harms nearly every organ of the body.
- Smoking causes heart disease and increases the risk of coronary heart disease by 2 to 4 times.
- Smoking increases the risk of stroke by 2 to 4 times.
- Smoking causes many diseases and reduces overall health.
- Smoking causes 90% of all lung cancer deaths and 80% of all deaths from chronic obstructive pulmonary disease.
- Smoking can cause cancer almost anywhere in your body.

♥ **Health Coach Wisdom:** You probably know someone who smokes; or you may smoke yourself. While quitting is difficult, many people are able to stop by getting help from a medical professional, through hypnosis and/or group support. It is possible to stop smoking and stopping can add years to your life.

Abusing your body by over doing exercise: People are often too hard on themselves when it comes to exercise. One of the worst things we do is to go for long periods of time without doing any activity and then go out and play or exercise too hard. Some people ski the high slopes, run 5 miles, and play racquetball or basketball after sitting all week. It is common for an out-of-condition person to throw out their back by swinging a golf club without warming up, or picking up a heavy object the wrong way. It happens too often. *We need to take time to warm up,* stay in good physical condition and stretch properly during the week. The best way to prevent an injury is to take time to get fit and then stay in good physical condition.

Risky Behavior: The topic of risky behavior covers everything from driving too fast, driving without a seat belt, texting while driving, driving or boating under the influence of alcohol or drugs, driving while tired, having unprotected sex with multiple partners, smoking, chewing tobacco or forgetting your sunscreen. This list goes on and on. Consider the consequences of your actions before you make risky choices. When accidents happen, they rarely affect only one person. That means your actions can change the course of your life and someone else's life—with decisions you make.

Abusing Alcohol and Other Mood Altering Substances

Alcohol is not a nutrient, it fact it is a member of a group of organic chemicals called ethanol. Physiologically, alcohol is a sedative and central nervous system depressant. Just like other drugs, the extent to which central nervous system function is impaired by alcohol consumption is directly related to the amount of alcohol in the blood. Similarly, like other drugs, any health benefits resulting from alcohol consumption depend on the amount of alcohol consumed.

Alcohol supplies energy to the body, in the form of 7 calories per gram. But unlike the other energy nutrients (carbohydrates, proteins and fats), alcohol is not an essential nutrient. In other words, it has no nutritional value. One downside comes from the additional calories provided by the alcohol, which may contribute to unwanted weight gain. A glass of wine daily can increase your weight by as much as ten pounds a year, unless you are physically active. On the positive side, studies have shown that moderate consumption, no more than 1 drink per day for women, and no more than one to two drinks per day for men may reduce the risk of heart disease. If you don't drink, don't start to protect your heart. There are many other ways to protect your heart health.

Impact of Alcohol

If you drink *excessively* on a regular basis, your nutritional status can become compromised. Protein deficiency can develop, both from the depression of protein synthesis in the cells and in the drinker who substitutes alcohol for food. Alcohol affects every tissue's nutrient metabolism in different ways:

- Stomach cells become inflamed and vulnerable to ulcers
- Intestinal cells fail to absorb thiamin, folate and vitamin B12
- Liver cells lose efficiency in activating vitamin D and become inflamed

- Rod cells in the retina which normally process Vitamin A alcohol (retinol) into the form needed for vision (retinal), process drinking alcohol instead
- Kidneys excrete increased quantities of magnesium, calcium, potassium, zinc and folate
- Causes vitamin B6 deficiency, lowering production of red blood cells

What is a Drink?

It doesn't matter what the beverage is, whether it is beer, wine, or a cocktail made with liquor, each serving contains the same amount of alcohol:

- 12 ounces of beer (150 calories)
- 5 ounces of wine (100 calories)
- 1 ½ ounces of 80-proof distilled spirits (100 calories)
- 12 ounce of bottled wine cooler (210-230 calories)
- 3 ounces of sherry or port (130 calories)
- 9 ¾ ounces of malt liquor (135 calories)

What is Binge Drinking?

Binge drinking is at least 5 drinks one at a time for men or 4 for women, in one sitting. The short term reactions caused by consuming large amounts of alcohol in a brief time are serious: vomiting, dizziness, impaired mental capabilities, risky sexual behavior *and even death*. *Does it happen often?*

> 50% of college men and 37% of college women report
> drinking more than 5 drinks at one sitting.

Alcohol and its Effects

Because alcohol is distributed so quickly and thoroughly in the body, it can affect the central nervous system, even in small concentrations. Even small amounts can slow reactions. Here is a list of effects to consider:

- **Alcohol and medication**–Use of prescription or over-the-counter medications can increase the effects of alcohol or may impair driving all on their own. Chronic, heavy drinking (*more than two drinks per day for women or more than four drinks per day for men*) appears to activate an enzyme that may be responsible for changing the over the counter pain reliever acetaminophen (Tylenol, for example) and many other others into chemicals that can **produce liver damage**.

- **Alcohol and hangovers**–A hangover is usually thought of as a group of ailments including: headache, nausea, vomiting, sensitivity to light and sound, dry mouth and irritability.
- **Alcohol and Driving**–NEVER DRINK AND DRIVE. Studies have shown that *even one drink* can considerably impair a driver's response time. Each year hundreds of thousands of people are injured and thousands die (*one alcohol related fatality every 31 minutes*) as a result of drunk driving.
- **Alcohol and Breast Cancer** –Even consumed in moderate amounts (one drink per day for women), alcohol may increase the risk of breast cancer in women.
- **Other cancers**–Heavy alcohol use, especially when combined with smoking, appears to increase risk of colon cancer and of the throat and esophagus. Risk of cancer increases for people with hepatitis and cirrhosis.
- **Liver Damage**–Alcoholic hepatitis (inflammation of the liver) and cirrhosis (scarring of liver tissue that interferes with blood flow and liver function) and hepatitis can lead to permanent liver damage if alcohol consumption continues.
- **High Blood Pressure and Stroke**–Heavy drinking is a major cause of high blood pressure, or hypertension, a risk factor for stroke and heart disease.
- **Night Blindness**–Alcohol blocks formation of retinal which is required for vision in low light.

Other ill effects of alcohol abuse include: brain damage, anemia, attacks of pancreatitis, irregular heartbeat, stroke, high blood pressure and emotional or social problems. Alcohol affects emotional centers in the limbic system, causing anxiety and depression. Emotional and physical effects of alcohol can contribute to marital and family problems including domestic violence and negative work related consequences.

What is Alcohol Abuse or Alcoholism?

Alcoholism is a dependency on alcohol characterized by craving, loss of control, physical dependence, withdrawal symptoms and tolerance. The following is a scale of alcohol addiction from Narcotics Anonymous (NA) and Alcoholics Anonymous (AA):

- **Use:** It is considered to be the ingestion of alcohol or other drugs without experiencing any negative consequences.
- **Misuse**: When a person experiences negative consequences from use of alcohol or other drugs, for example: receiving a DUI or being in an automobile accident.

- **Abuse**: Abuse constitutes continued use of alcohol or other drugs in spite of negative consequences. If a person does not have a substance abuse problem, they will be able to cut back on their alcohol consumption or give it up after a negative consequence, such as a DUI. *People who continue to drink and drive abuse alcohol.*
- **Dependency/Addiction**: Compulsive use of alcohol or other drugs, regardless of adverse or negative consequences, presents the problem of dependency or addiction. Such individuals should seek professional help to stop the progression.
- **Alcoholics Anonymous (AA)** is perhaps the most well known program to deal with alcohol addiction. This not for profit organization, established in 1935, has helped millions of people to deal with this life altering disease. *Their "12-Step Program" focuses not only on the physical act of abstaining from alcohol, but the psychosocial aspects as well.*

Alcohol mixed with prescription or other drugs can have dangerous consequences such as nausea, vomiting, headache, mental impairment, risk of heart attack, liver damage, stomach bleeding and death by overdose—to name a few. If you are on medications, consult your physician regarding the interactions with alcohol.

Anyone who has a relationship with someone who has a problem with alcohol or drug addiction knows that recommending that your loved one "get help" is not usually well received. Getting emotional support for yourself is the best thing to do. Your reactions can make the problem worse or you can take the lead by getting help.

Abuse of prescription drugs is a crisis in America. Physicians are prescribing addictive pain killers at an alarming rate. Deaths from drug overdose have been steadily rising over the past two decades and have become the leading cause of injury death in the United States. The drug overdose death rate more than doubled from 1999 to 2013. Americans consume 80 percent of the opiate painkillers produced in the world, according to the American Society of Interventional Pain Physicians. Every hour a baby is born in the U.S. with symptoms of opiate withdrawal, according to a study published in April by the Journal of the American Medical Association.

A record 4.02 billion drug prescriptions were written in the U.S. in 2011, says the journal ACS Chemical Neuroscience.

We take a pill for everything. Adding to the problem are doctors who are prescribing drugs for depression without physiological or psychological counseling or follow-up. Doctors are too busy to take time to get to the root cause. We are becoming a society of people who wants to take a pill to solve our problems, when more often the prescription for what we need is to heal holistically through good health habits and support. If you or someone you know needs help with addiction, please review the resources listed at the end of this chapter. Reach out. There are compassionate, trusted, knowledgeable people that can help you bring light to a dark situation.

♥ **Health Coach Wisdom:** Inside each of us is a tremendous amount of wisdom. We need to meditate to connect with our higher self. When our mind is at peace we have a greater awareness of ourselves and no longer feel the need to medicate our anxiousness. Meditation can help overcome addictions to drinking, drugs, gambling, shopping, overeating, or smoking.

Stay on your recovery path, ask for help, when you need it and
never despair, for there is a way through every block.
~ Tommy Rosen, Recovery 2.0

Affirmation to quit smoking or change an unwanted behavior:

I decide what is best for my body and I am eager to make positive changes.

My Action Steps

Take time to think about how you will change your health for the better. Nothing will change unless you do something different. Take action today by listing three steps you will take to move out of your comfort zone and move toward a brighter tomorrow. *Consider the following questions:*

Who will you reach out to? What resources will you seek? What steps will you take to sleep better and prevent illness or injury? What area of your health needs attention?

- _____
- _____
- _____

Helping and loving others fills your world with love.
~Erik Olesen, author *Mastering the Winds of Change*

Books and Resources:

Recovery 2.0–Move Beyond Addiction and Upgrade your Life, www.tommyrosen.com

www.SAMHSA.GOV. Substance Abuse and Mental Health Services Administration whose mission is to reduce the impact of substance abuse in America's communities. 1-877-726-4727.

Spirit Junkie~A Radical Road to Self-Love and Miracles by Gabrielle Bernstein, 2011.

Intervention–How to Help Someone Who Doesn't Want Help–A Step by Step Guide for Families and Friends of Chemically Dependent Persons. By Vernon E. Johnson, D.D. by Hazelden Foundation. 1986.

The Alcoholism and Addiction Cure–A Holistic Approach to Total Recovery by Chris Prentiss, Power Publishing, 2007. www.passagesmalibu.com.

Chopra Center for Wellbeing, www.chopra.com/freedom or call 888-424-6772.

Alcoholics Anonymous: www.aa.org. Al-Anon. Strength and hope for families and friends of problem drinkers. www.al-anon.alateen.org.

www.helpguide.org. A trusted non-profit resource. Your guide to better mental health.

www.smokefree.gov. For help to quit smoking.

Partnership for Drug Free Kids. www.drugfree.org.

Chapter 9

Secrets of Healthy Cooking

Focus on the Foods You Love

Eating nourishing food that you love is the foundation of great health. Meal planning is the key to eating nutritious foods. Some people perceive meal planning as difficult. It isn't. You just need a simple strategy and some ideas. Taking a few minutes each week to plan your meals is easy and it takes away the stress of wondering what you are going to eat. I love to plan meals, shop for new and different ingredients and entertain friends and family with wholesome meals. It is also fun to find new restaurants that take pride in serving fresh and flavorful cuisine.

Planning your meals is also key to reaching and maintaining a healthy weight when you focus on what *you can eat*, not what you can't. *Tell yourself that you can have anything, so you never feel deprived or activate your food radar looking for things you "shouldn't" have.* Focus on delicious, healthy, and fresh foods that make you happy.

Treat yourself to foods like sweet blueberries, flavorful homegrown tomatoes, toasted almonds, walnuts, freshly grated parmesan cheese, creamy yogurt, crisp apples, grilled wild salmon, butternut squash, and homemade whole grain breads. Sometimes only comfort foods will do, so I have found a way to make these more nutritious with less calories and fat. When you prepare your own salad dressings, soups and meals, you can use fresh ingredients and will eat less processed food that can have unhealthy additives. People are always asking me for ideas on what to eat, as it has been my lifelong passion to eat and prepare delicious food. In this chapter, you'll find easy ideas on how to lighten up traditional dishes. Chapter 10 has easy recipes for two week's worth of nutritious breakfasts, lunches, dinners, snacks, and desserts.

♥ **Health Coach Wisdom:** The key to healthy eating is to simplify your meal planning, shopping and meal preparation while getting the most nutrition possible.

It was my goal to create a recipe book of lighter favorite meals and snacks to simplify eating well. *You can adapt them to your taste.* They say cooking is an art, while baking is a science. This means baking is very exact–that the recipe should be followed precisely. In contrast, when you are preparing things like soups, salads, sandwiches and casseroles you can change the recipe to add or leave out ingredients as you wish. If you like your food spicy, then add more spices. If you don't like walnuts, switch to almonds. If you are a vegetarian, leave out the meat and replace it with vegetable protein, tofu or beans. Read labels and choose foods with natural ingredients. Make cooking your own; make your meals with love and with the intention that you have the *power to be healthy.*

Meal Planning

On my website you can download a free simple meal planning form, titled *This Week's Menus.* I have been using this tool for years as a way to take the stress out of deciding what to eat each day. The method is simple:

1. Check your calendar and plan your meals around weekly activities
2. Plan which days you will cook, pick up dinner or eat out depending on your schedule.
3. For days you will be home in time to make dinner, find ideas in your favorite cookbooks, magazines or online. Selecting foods that are in season will taste better and help you save money. Use your slow cooker when you won't be home early enough to cook. You don't have to plan out your breakfasts, lunches and dinners for every day. However, if you write down even a few meals, then you can *make your grocery list* to make sure you have everything you need on hand when you begin to prepare your meals. *Having fresh, flavorful ingredients in your house is the key to eating well!*
4. For each meal, aim to eat from the food groups, including a fruit and/or vegetable, grain, lean protein, nuts or legumes and dairy. *Choose foods that work best for you.* Eating a variety of foods from each group is the key to getting needed nutrients, fiber, vitamins and minerals.

♥ **Health Coach Wisdom:** When you know what you are going to have for lunch and dinner, your day will go more smoothly, your meals will taste better and you will feel better. *When I forget to make my weekly meal plan, it creates stress, bad tasting meals and a lack of nutrition.*

Anyone can cook, and most everyone should.
– Mark Bittman, author of *How to Cook Everything*

How to Make Recipes Healthier

Most of your favorite recipes can be easily changed to lower the sugar, saturated fat, sodium and calories while you increase vegetables, fruits and fiber. You can use the following tips to help you create your own healthier recipes:

Key # 1: Cut the Saturated Fat

- Replace high fat meat with a leaner, lower-fat meat or vegetarian alternative. If a recipe calls for ground beef, use extra–lean ground beef, lean ground turkey breast or soy crumbles.
- Make the portion size smaller. Aim for no more than 3 ounces per serving.
- If you use a fattier cut of meat, after it is cooked, drain off all the fat and then season it with herbs, seasonings and vegetables like onions, peppers and garlic.
- Grill, broil, stir-fry or roast your meat, fish and chicken and never deep fry.

Key # 2: Lower the Amount of Sugar, Saturated Fat and Calories

- Look at each recipe for ways you can reduce the fat and cut the sugar or calories.
- You can usually cut back on sugar in recipes by one third to one half. Add more spices, such as cinnamon and nutmeg, or flavorings such as vanilla.
- Fats, oil, butter or margarines, can usually be cut by one-third to one-half in recipes. Experiment so that you still have flavor, but not excess fat and calories.
- To replace the moisture and flavor lost when fat is reduced, you can make up the difference with broth, wine, fat-free milk, soy or almond milk, flax meal, fruit juice, and extra herbs, spices and vegetables.
- For a moist baked product when fat is reduced, substitute with dried fruits, applesauce, prune butter or flax meal.
- Replace high fat dairy products such as cream with low-fat or fat-free versions.
- Use correct portions of high calorie foods, such as avocados, coconut, cheese and nuts. (*Healthy foods can still be high in calories and fat. Know your portions.*)

Key # 3: Increase the Vegetables, Fruits and Fiber

- Add frozen, fresh or precut vegetables
- Add frozen, canned or fresh fruits

- Use whole grains for all or part of the recipe
- When possible, leave skins on fruits or vegetables (wash thoroughly)
- Add beans to soups and salads and serve as a side dish more often
- Grate or finely chop vegetables such as zucchini, onions, celery, carrots, tomatoes, spinach, or any vegetables and add to sauces or casseroles. Any time you can add extra vegetables, do so!

A New Way to Think About Cooking

I was having lunch with a young college student who proudly exclaimed, "I don't cook!" She said it as if she was proving something. I know a lot of people who are proud of the fact that they don't cook or say they don't like to cook. For those who think cooking is a lot of trouble or fear making mistakes, I offer the following perspective on cooking:

Cooking does not have to be difficult or time consuming. In fact, most of the foods we consume during the day don't even have to be cooked, just assembled. Following a recipe is the easiest way to learn to cook. Meals can be prepared easily if you have the right ingredients on hand. Remember you are the one who decides what foods are going into your body. If you love to eat good tasting, quality food, then you will be rewarded when you learn how to prepare delicious food. You control the quality, the taste, the calories, sugar, fat and sodium when you make it yourself.

Most people are so busy with the details of their lives that they leave out the one thing that will assure them a healthy, delicious meal—they fail to plan. The key to eating great food is planning in advance, shopping and storing it properly, so that when you walk in the door from a busy day, you have a plan of action. You will be able to whip up something wonderful to eat in no time.

Fine Food Fast

Here are a few tips for eating well:

- Make a weekly meal plan by getting ideas from books, magazines and the internet. There are sites that even create your shopping lists for you!
- Plan quicker recipes for busy days, including slow cooker and grilled recipes.
- Look for recipes that are low in saturated fats, sodium, and sugar.
- When planning for your week, look for ways to incorporate using food from one meal into a second meal to speed up prep time.

- ♥ Create a weekly shopping list
- ♥ Be flexible when shopping to include in-season produce or sale items
- ♥ When you get home from the grocery store, wash and pre-cut produce
- ♥ Ask for help from family members with putting groceries away, chopping, mixing or stirring, setting the table and doing dishes. Get the whole family involved. Make it fun! Cooking and sharing food brings people together.
- ♥ When cooking for one meal, think ahead and do things like grilling extra chicken breasts for another meal. Cut up carrots, celery, onions, or peppers, chop or slice extras and pre-bag them for snacks or cooking.
- ♥ Add fresh ingredients as often as possible!

Common Problems and Easy Solutions

When working with clients, I often hear the same complaints. People get stuck on the problem and develop a belief that keeps them from developing healthy eating habits. Here are some simple solutions to common problems:

Problem: "I find it hard to eat the daily recommendation of vegetables."

Solution: First make it your intention to eat more vegetables. Add a vegetable to each meal and snack. For example: Sauté vegetables like spinach, green onions and bell peppers in an egg scramble for breakfast. Choose soup and/or salad for lunch. At the salad bar add in as many fresh vegetables as possible and cut back on the high calorie toppings like cheese and salad dressing. Have carrots, snap peas, celery, and cherry tomatoes with whole grain crackers and humus for your afternoon snack. For dinner always have a side vegetable along with soup or salad and add veggies to you main dish. One or more days of the week, serve a vegetarian meal as your main entrée. If you follow this method you will get the proper number of servings each day.

Problem: "I live alone and don't want to cook for myself."

Solution: Treat yourself like someone you love. We take the time to prepare meals for others, and you deserve the same special treatment. You can keep it simple, and by shopping for fresh, whole foods and having them on hand you will be able to put together easy meals. Make a pot of soup or other favorite dishes and freeze them in small portions to pull out for quick meals. Swap half your recipe with a friend for variety. You'll be helping them too.

Problem: "I let food go bad and I waste a lot of money."

Solution: Make a weekly meal plan and stick to it. You can switch days around if something unexpected comes up, but at least you will have the food you need on hand to make nutritious meals. **Don't plan every meal of the week,** just pick three or four days that you will make dinner. Eat leftover food for lunch or use for another meal. When you know what meal you are going to use your cauliflower for, it won't go to waste. **Wash and chop veggies ahead of time** and store in containers in your refrigerator to speed up your cooking time.

Problem: "I don't like vegetables."

Solution: **Experiment with new ways to prepare veggies**: Season with herbs and spices and roast, grill or stir fry them to bring out the best flavor.

Learn about the benefits of eating vegetables and you will be more motivated to eat them. For example, why are leafy greens so important? Greens are believed to be good for your heart, thanks to the folate (vitamin B9) they contain. Research shows that getting 400 micrograms of folate a day can lower homocysteine-*an amino acid that in too high amounts may be a risk factor for heart disease.* Leafy greens, romaine lettuce, Brussels sprouts, avocado, spinach, broccoli and mustard greens are all high in folate. Add these to your mixed salad greens and soups. Toss into a stir fry or steam and serve as a quick side dish. You gain the fiber, minerals and vitamins essential to good health.

♥ **Health Coach Wisdom:** We need to eat a variety of foods from different groups to get the nutrients we need. For example, lentils, beans and oranges also contain Vitamin B-9 or folate. Oranges, kiwis and bell peppers are high in Vitamin C. The easiest way to get the vitamins, minerals and nutrients you need is to eat a wide variety of foods in each group. Choose different colors which provide different benefits. *That is why nutritionists say "Eat a rainbow of colors."*

♥ **Fill your kitchen with healthy, delicious and life giving foods and you will always be ready for your next meal.** Visit your local farmer's market and talk to the farmers. You won't find a friendlier group of people to answer your questions and provide you with the freshest, best tasting foods you have ever eaten. We need to support our farmers.

Well Stocked Kitchen

Pantry

- **Beans**: kidney, garbanzo, black beans, pinto beans, refried beans (no fat), white navy beans, vegetarian chili, turkey chili, black eyed peas
- **Canned tomatoes:** diced, whole, crushed
- **Sun dried tomatoes**, artichoke hearts, water chestnuts
- **Soups:** low sodium soups, chicken broth, vegetable broth–*no msg*
- **Peanut butter**: Organic. no hydrogenated oils, almond butter
- **Hot cereal**: oatmeal–slow cooking, quick cooking and steel cut
- **Cold cereals**: 3 grams of fiber or more: Kashi Go Lean, Shredded Wheat, Bran Flakes, etc. Look for whole grains and less than 4-8 grams of sugar.
- **Canned fish:** light tuna in water, canned shrimp, crab, and salmon
- **Crackers:** multi-grain with no trans fats, pretzels, popcorn (no fat)
- **Protein bars**: Read labels, no trans fats, low sugar, least processed.
- **Dried fruits**: raisins, cranberries, blueberries, prunes, etc.
- **Canned** fruit: mandarins, pears, peaches and pineapple
- **Pasta:** Whole grains. Try Barilla Pasta Plus with extra fiber & protein
- **Pasta sauces:** Aim for lower sodium and saturated fat, less than 2 grams
- **Bragg** Liquid Aminos, apple cider vinegar, low sodium soy sauce
- **Potatoes:** Russet, red, Yukon gold, fingerling
- **Onions (**white, red, yellow)/ **garlic**
- **Fresh fruit:** bananas, oranges, apples, grapes, pineapple, kiwi, melons, papaya, mangoes, strawberries, raspberries, blueberries, melons, peaches, apricots
- **Drinks:** Fruit juices, soy milk, almond milk, water, tea, coffee
- **Oils:** extra virgin olive oil, canola oil, cooking spray
- **Bread:** whole grains (at least 2 or more grams of fiber)
- **Tortillas and pitas**: whole grain

Baking

- **Flours:** Whole wheat flour, whole grain oat, rye, almond, corn meal *(refrigerated)*
- **Baking soda**, **baking powder**, corn starch
- **Sweeteners**: sugar, brown sugar, agave sweetener, honey

Freezer

- **Meats:** Organic boneless, skinless chicken breasts, pork chops, lean ground turkey, lean ground beef & chicken
- **Frozen fish**: wild salmon, halibut, tilapia, scallops, shrimp
- **Vegetarian**: "sausage patties, chicken-less patties, burgers"
- **Frozen fruits:** blueberries, strawberries, mixed berries, peaches, etc.
- **Vegetables**: peas, corn, mixed vegetables, broccoli, cauliflower, peppers, stir fry mixes with green beans, mushrooms, edamame (soy), snow peas
- **Light ice cream**, **frozen yogurt:** Fat-free or low-fat
- **Waffles** or pancake mix: multigrain (keep refrigerated)
- **Frozen meals** with sodium less than 700 mg and no partially hydrogenated oils, vegetarian and vegan entrees

Spice Cupboard

- Salt & pepper, Mrs. Dash and other no-salt seasonings
- Italian seasoning, basil, oregano, thyme, cinnamon, nutmeg, chili powder
- Dry mustard, curry powder, cumin, spice rubs, garlic & herb powder
- Old Bay Seasoning for fish, Bell's seasoning for poultry

Refrigerator - *Keep your refrigerator set at 35-40 degrees*

- **Milk**: Fat-free or 1%, soy milk, almond milk, cashew milk, rice milk
- **Dairy:** Fat-free or low-fat sour cream
- **Yogurts:** plain, fat-free or low-fat, look for lower sugar
- **Cottage cheese,** low-fat or fat-free, low-fat cream cheese
- **Eggs** and liquid egg substitute (made from egg whites)
- **Butter** and/or other healthy butter spreads *–no partially hydrogenated oil*
- **Cheese**: cheddar cheese, fresh parmesan cheese, feta cheese
- **Roasted deli meats:** roasted lean turkey and ham – ***no nitrates***
- **Vinegars** for dressings, sun dried tomatoes, cherry peppers, wax peppers
- **Condiments**: low sugar jam, mustards, ketchup, soy sauce, teriyaki, horseradish, light mayonnaise such as Smart Beat or Best Foods Light
- **Fruit Juices**: 100%
- **Produce**: carrots, celery, lettuce, green onion, radishes, broccoli, asparagus, peppers, cauliflower, leafy greens such as spinach, kale, bok choy, Swiss chard, lettuce, cabbage, Brussels sprouts, mushrooms, squash, pumpkin, sweet potatoes, green beans, artichokes
- **Herbs**: Jar of minced garlic, tubes of herbs such as basil, parsley, ginger
- **Tortillas**: 100% Whole grain tortillas, 100% whole grain bread

- **Wheat Germ, flax meal** for cereals, and baking
- **Grains**: brown rice, wild rice, barley, bulgur, quinoa, couscous, farro, polenta
- **Nuts**: Walnuts, almonds, pecans, cashews, peanuts, brazil nuts, pistachios
- **Nut butters**: peanut, cashew, sunflower seed, almond butters
- **Bouillon:** jar of chicken, beef, vegetable or vegetarian seasonings
- **Meats:** should be 90% lean, fish, poultry, pork, beef
- **Tofu/ Miso**

You will notice in the following recipes that I mention some name brand items such as Earth Balance or Smart Balance Buttery Spreads, Bragg Apple Cider Vinegar, Liquid Aminos, Stonyfield Organic Yogurts, Mrs. Dash seasonings and others. I am always on the lookout for items that I can use to add flavor while reducing the saturated fat in my recipes. These products all taste excellent and as far as I have found, are good choices for preparing healthy meals. I love hearing about new food items that make healthy eating easier. If you have any healthy recipes or food products you would like to share with me, please send me an e-mail or contact me through my website at www.lynellross.com.

May you always enjoy great food and a healthy, happy life!

Cooking for yourself is the only sure way to take back control of your diet from the food scientists and food processors, and to guarantee you're eating real food and not edible foodlike substances…Not surprisingly, the decline in home cooking closely parallels the rise in obesity, and research suggests that people who cook are more likely to eat a more healthful diet.
Michael Pollan, *Food Rules, An Eater's Manual*

Books and Resources for Healthy Cooking:

How to Cook Everything, Simple Recipes for Great Food by Mark Bittman, Macmillan, 1998.
Quick & Easy Cookbook
Over 200 Healthful Recipes You Can Prepare in Minutes by The American Heart Association.
Placer County Real Food from Farmers Markets, Recipes & Menus for every week of the year by Joanne Neft and Laura Kenny, 2010.
Everyday Food Light-The Quickest and Easiest Recipes All Under 500 Calories, 2011 by Martha Stewart Living Omnimedia, Inc.
Eating Well Magazine- www.eatingwell.com for healthy cooking tips, meal planning ideas.
*Cooking Light Magazine-*www.cookinglight.com for healthy cooking tips, snacks and more.
Crazy Sexy Kitchen-150 Plant –Empowered Recipes to ignite a mouthwatering revolution by Kris Carr with Chef Chad Sarno, Hay House Inc., 2012.

Chapter 10

Recipes for a Healthy Life

The following recipes are for simple comfort foods. My goal was to develop healthy, everyday meals and snacks and to provide you with nutritional information so you can keep track of and understand more about the foods you eat. It took me years to develop these recipes. I started by finding dishes from friends, relatives, cookbooks, on-line websites and magazines, and then I experimented with them by reducing the fat, sugar and sodium. It wasn't always pretty. In fact, my husband and sons had to eat some tasteless meals. However, with practice, taking classes, reading and asking questions, I learned how to make everyday recipes healthier and better tasting.

In the process, I learned that you can save a lot of calories, fat, sugar and salt by simply cutting back on the amounts you use. For example, you can serve a taco with one ounce of cheddar cheese, but if you add only *one more ounce*—you add an additional 9 grams of fat. Every extra tablespoon of oil, butter, or mayonnaise adds 12 grams of fat. *Our bodies simply do not need large amounts of fat, salt and sugar, especially at one meal.*

I used a computer program for every recipe typing in the ingredients to get the nutritional values and information. *You will see the nutritional information on each recipe, together with the serving size and number of servings from each food group.* I did this so you can keep track of the nutrition you are getting every day. Aim to eat from the food groups each day, and cut back where you can reduce the overall amounts of fat, sugar, and sodium. Enhance the flavor and texture of food with herbs, spices and cooking methods. The important thing for you to remember is that every serving you eat doubles the amount of calories, fat, carbohydrates and everything. That is all right as long as you are aware of your daily totals. Knowing and remembering what you eat is your key to getting the best nutrition and staying within your healthy body weight range.

Fresh, whole foods do not need to be drowning in butter, deep fried or coated in sugar to taste good. We need to regain our taste for fresh foods and listen to what our bodies need. My hope in developing these recipes is to provide you with everyday foods that you can enjoy while you begin to create your own healthy lifestyle and recipes you love.

Breakfasts Too Good to Skip

~

Green Power Smoothie

The morning is no time to skip meals. Making a smoothie is the quickest way to get powerful nutrition. Keep fresh ingredients on hand for a fast breakfast.

1 cup spinach or kale washed and stripped off the stocks.
½ cup pineapple
½ cup light soy milk

1 cup green tea, chilled
1 tablespoon flax meal
½ banana, sliced
2 Tablespoons protein powder.

1. Mix all ingredients in your blender and go.

Servings: 1

Nutrition Facts: Amount Per Serving: Calories 312, Total Fat 7g, Saturated Fat <1g, Cholesterol 0, Sodium 87mg, Potassium 644mg, Total Carbohydrates 37g, Fiber 9g, Sugar 32g, Protein 16g

Food Group Servings: 1 vegetable, 2 fruit,

Health Coach Tips:
- ♥ When you have bananas that begin to over ripen, peel, wrap in plastic wrap and freeze them individually. Take them out of the freezer and cut into chunks to add to your smoothies. They add valuable potassium and make your smoothies cool and creamy.
- ♥ Add more green vegetables to your day by starting in the morning adding spinach, kale or Swiss chard to your smoothies. Leafy greens increase your energy, may help regulate blood sugar and are a prime source of antioxidants and vitamins.
- ♥ Pineapple has vitamin C, an antioxidant that helps with immune health, and protects against heart disease and infections, especially important for people with diabetes.

Health Coach Energy Smoothie

I used to think I would prefer to eat my foods whole, but when I am pressed for time, making a smoothie provides me with a quick way to pack in lots of vital nutrients from fruits, vegetables and protein. I make a different flavor every day and I never get tired of them. *Try having a smoothie everyday for a week. Put in whatever you like and see how much better you feel!*

1 medium banana, peeled and sliced
½ cup orange juice or 1 whole orange
    peeled or any fruit you like
1 cup fat-free milk, light soy milk, or
    almond milk

½ cup yogurt, plain, fat-free
3 tablespoons isolated whey protein
    powder, vanilla
½ cup crushed ice

1. Place all ingredients in blender and mix until smooth and fluffy. Enjoy!

Servings: 2

Per Serving: Serving size: ½ the recipe (13.1 oz), 250 calories, fat 4g, cholesterol 21mg, sodium 131mg, carbohydrates 35 g, fiber 3g, sugar 22g, protein 19g

Food Group Servings: 2 fruit, 1.5 dairy

Health Coach Tips:
♥ The amino acids in the protein powder have been proven to help improve your mood as does the banana which increases the serotonin in your brain, helping you to feel calmer and happier.
♥ Select a whey protein powder that is low in sugar. Sugar spikes your energy for a time, but quickly crashes your blood sugar levels leaving you feeling irritated and shaky. Having a small amount of protein with each meal or snack keeps your blood sugar levels even keel. *Be sure to count the number of calories in the type of protein powder you choose.*
♥ You can substitute any fruit for the banana and you do not have to add the orange juice if you want to cut down on the sugar-*even though real orange juice provides natural sugar.* Oranges provide vitamin C, folate and potassium to slow heart and gum disease and helps prevent you from getting sick.

Breakfast Veggie Scramble

You can choose to use whole eggs or egg substitute, which is made of egg whites, and has less cholesterol. Optional additions or toppers include avocado slices, salsa, or grated cheddar cheese. Just be sure to be aware of the extra calories and fats. *You always have the control over how much and what you eat.*

¾ cup egg substitute (equal to 3 eggs)
3 green onions, chopped
1 green pepper, chopped
¼ cup green chilies, chopped
¼ cup fat-free sour cream or plain yogurt

1 tomato diced
1 tablespoon canola oil
1 tablespoon butter
¼ cup onions, white or red

1. In a large nonstick skillet, on medium heat, sauté onions, peppers, and chilies in 1 tablespoon canola oil until slightly soft.
2. Push veggies to the sides and add 1 tablespoon of butter or healthy type margarine and pour in liquid egg substitute. Gently fold veggies into the egg mixture and let brown slightly on the bottom while stirring occasionally.
3. When cooked to set, place egg mixture on plates. Top with chopped tomato and sour cream.

Servings: 2

Nutrition Facts: Serving size: ½ of a recipe (12.5 ounces), Amount Per Serving: Calories 185, Total Fat 9g, Saturated Fat 3g, Cholesterol 10mg, Sodium 309mg, Potassium 770mg, Total Carbohydrates 13g, Fiber 3g, Sugar 7g, Protein 13g

Food Group Servings: 1 eggs/protein group, 2 vegetable, 1 fat

Heavenly Carrot Muffins

Compared to many restaurant carrot cakes and muffins, which have double and even triple the amount of fat and calories, these healthful carrot muffins will satisfy you as a quick breakfast with a yogurt or piece of fruit. Also perfect for a midmorning snack.

¾ cup whole wheat flour

1 cup all-purpose flour

1 teaspoon baking soda

½ teaspoon baking powder

Pinch of salt

1 teaspoon cinnamon

2 egg whites, slightly beaten

⅓ cup honey

2 tablespoons canola oil

2 tablespoons golden flax meal

¼ cup orange juice

¼ cup nonfat plain yogurt

1 teaspoon vanilla extract

Grated zest of ½ orange

1 cup grated carrots

½ cup raisins or golden currants

¾ cup chopped walnuts or pecans

¼ cup applesauce, unsweetened

1. Preheat the oven to 350 degrees. Spray a 12 slot muffin tin with cooking spray, add cupcake liners, and spray those.
2. Over a large bowl, put a large metal strainer. Add the flours, baking soda, baking powder, salt, and cinnamon. Shake the flour contents until they sift through to the bowl. Add the raisins and stir in with a fork to coat.
3. In a large mixing bowl, beat the eggs and honey until well mixed. Beat in the oil, juice, yogurt, vanilla, and grated zest.
4. Add the dry ingredients, and then fold in the carrot and nuts. Beat by hand until well mixed.
5. Pour the batter into the prepared tins and bake for 20 to 25 minutes or until golden brown. Cool on rack.

Serving: 1

Nutrition Facts: Serving size: Makes 12, 2.6 ounce muffins. Amount Per Serving: Calories 204, Total Fat 8.g, Saturated Fat 0.71g, Cholesterol 0.31mg, Sodium 146mg, Potassium 169mg, Total Carbohydrates 29g, Fiber 1.68g, Sugar 11g, Protein 5g

Food Group Servings: 1 grain, ¼ serving fruit, 1.5 fat

Health Coach Tip:
- Slice your carrot muffin in half and spread with low-fat cream cheese or almond butter for a satisfying snack.

199

Low-Fat Apple Butter Bran Muffins

You make these low in fat by replacing butter or oil with apple butter and using egg whites. Muffins from the grocery store are usually loaded with partially hydrogenated soybean oil and trans fats which are the worst thing you can consume for heart health.

1 cup whole wheat flour	1 cup apple butter
1 cup all-bran cereal	1 cup buttermilk, low-fat
½ cup oat bran	2 egg whites
1 teaspoon baking soda	½ cup raisins (optional)
½ teaspoon cinnamon	

1. Combine the flour, bran cereal, oat bran, baking soda and cinnamon and stir well. Do not over mix. Add the apple butter, buttermilk, and egg whites and stir just until the dry ingredients are moistened. Fold in the raisins.
2. Coat muffin cups with cooking spray, and fill ¾ full with batter. Bake for 15 to 18 minutes or until a wooden toothpick comes out clean.
3. Remove from muffin tin after they have been out of the oven for about 5 minutes.

Servings: 12

Nutrition Facts: Serving size: ¹⁄₁₂ of a recipe (2.9 ounces), Amount Per Serving: Calories 131, Total Fat 0.71g, Saturated Fat 0.2g, Cholesterol 0.82mg, Sodium 171mg, Potassium 231mg, Total Carbohydrates 30.5g, Fiber 4.2g, Sugar 15g, Protein 4g

Food Group Servings: 1.5 grain

Egg Muffin Powerhouse

Faster than a drive thru, more powerful than a white flour, high fat breakfast sandwich, you make this one tastier, and better for you. Packed with protein, vegetables, and fiber, this will stay with you throughout the morning.

1 double fiber English muffin

2 egg whites, lightly beaten

1 tablespoon Parmesan cheese
    freshly grated

2 tomato slices

2 tablespoons green pepper chopped

1 tablespoon Smart Balance or
    Earth Balance

1. Toast your whole grain or whole wheat English muffin.
2. Melt 1 teaspoon margarine in skillet, sauté your veggies for 1 or 2 minutes, then add your egg whites.
3. Cook on one side until golden brown, flip over egg mixture, and sprinkle on your cheese. Cook on medium until egg is done and cheese is melted, one or two minutes. Cut into pieces that will fit on your muffin.
4. Spread remaining margarine on muffin, and then add egg mixture. Wrap in parchment paper and go!

Servings: 2

Nutrition Facts: Serving size: 1(18.5ounces), Amount Per Serving: Calories 300, Total Fat 7g, Saturated Fat 3g, Cholesterol 8.8mg, Sodium 570 mg, Potassium 798mg, Total Carbohydrates 42g, Fiber 9g, Sugar 15g, Protein 21g

Food Group Servings: 2 grain, 1 protein/egg, 1 vegetable, 1 fat

Health Coach Tip:
♥ You can choose to use freshly washed baby spinach, chopped bell pepper, chopped green chilies, sliced green onions or any veggies you have on hand. The more vegetables you use, the more taste and nutrition.

Multigrain Pancakes with Homemade Berry Syrup

I make a batch of these on Sunday mornings instead of plain pancakes with sugary syrup. These hearty, healthy pancakes add healthy protein and fiber that keeps everyone full until lunch! For smaller appetites and less carbohydrates, eat two pancakes with a yogurt topping.

1 ½ cup whole wheat flour	2 tablespoons sugar
1 cup unbleached all-purpose flour	3 eggs
1 cup oats	¼ cup pecans, chopped
½ cup cornmeal	2 tablespoons flax meal
1 teaspoon baking powder	2 tablespoons canola oil
2 teaspoons baking soda	3 cups fresh or frozen blueberries or mixed berries
1 teaspoon salt	2 tablespoons cornstarch
4 cups low-fat (1%) buttermilk	⅓ cup no sugar, all fruit jam

1. In a large mixing bowl combine whole wheat flour, all-purpose flour, oats, corn meal, baking powder, baking soda and salt; mix well.
2. Beat eggs in a bowl with buttermilk, add in sugar and stir until blended.
3. Slowly add buttermilk mixture to the flour mixture, blending well. Fold in nuts.
4. **To make syrup**: In a medium saucepan, stir together berries and jam. In a small bowl, stir together 1 tablespoon of cornstarch and two tablespoons water. Mix until blended. Slowly add to berry mixture and heat until boiling for one minute. Mixture will thicken. Keep warm until you serve pancakes.
5. Heat skillet and spray with nonstick spray. Ladle batter into skillet heated to 350 degrees using a ⅓ cup measure. Cook until golden brown on both sides.

Servings: 9 (3 pancakes per serving)

Nutrition Facts: Serving size: ⅑ of a recipe (8.7 ounces), Amount Per Serving: Calories 388, Total Fat 10g, Saturated Fat 2g, Cholesterol 75mg, Sodium 735mg, Potassium 368mg, Total Carbohydrates 61g, Fiber 5g, Sugar 13g, Protein 14g

Food Group Servings: 2 grain, 1 dairy, 1 fruit, 1fat

Health Coach Tips:
- This recipe makes 28 pancakes. If you do not eat them all, wrap individually in plastic and freeze. When you are in a hurry, pop them in the toaster for a quick and delicious breakfast on week days. Serve with yogurt and fruit for a well balanced breakfast.
- Create your own favorite combinations: Bananas and walnuts or finely diced apples and cinnamon. What is your favorite fruit?

Oat & Berry Breakfast Bars

These moist bars make a great on the go breakfast or snack with a glass of milk and an apple.

2 cups oats
1 cup whole wheat flour
1 cup pecans, chopped
6 ounces raspberries
4 ounces dried blueberries

¼ cup honey
½ cup brown sugar
¼ cup Smart Balance
1 teaspoon baking soda
2 eggs, lightly beaten

1. Preheat oven to 350 degrees and spray a 9 x 13 pan with cooking spray.
2. Combine oats, flour, pecans, raspberries, and blueberries in a large bowl.
3. Combine honey, brown sugar, Smart Balance, baking soda, and eggs in a small bowl. Stir into the oat mixture until well mixed.
4. Spread into the prepared pan and bake for 25 minutes.
5. Let cool and cut into 16 bars for breakfast or 20 smaller squares for snacks.

Servings: 16

Nutrition Facts: Serving size: ¹⁄₁₆ of a recipe (3.5 ounces), Amount Per Serving: Calories 236, Total Fat 8g, Saturated Fat 1g, Cholesterol 26mg, Sodium 111mg, Potassium 202mg, Total Carbohydrates 36g, Fiber 5g, Sugar 15g, Protein 7g

Food Group Servings: 1 grain, ½ nuts, 1 fat

Oven Baked Apple Cinnamon French Toast

Make this the night before to serve an easy hot breakfast in the morning!

12 slices day old multigrain bread
3 eggs, lightly beaten
3 egg whites, lightly beaten
1 ½ cups 1% milk
2 tablespoons sugar

1 teaspoon vanilla
⅛ teaspoon salt
2 teaspoons cinnamon
1 teaspoon lemon juice
3 cups chopped apples, washed and diced with peels

1. Spray a 9 x 13 baking pan with cooking spray. Cut bread into cubes and put into a large mixing bowl.
2. In a medium bowl beat eggs, whisk in milk, 1 tablespoon of sugar, vanilla and salt. Pour egg mixture over bread cubes.
3. Chop the apples, toss with 1 teaspoon of lemon juice. Add apples to the egg and bread mixture and toss to coat. Pour the mixture into your prepared pan and refrigerate overnight.
4. In the morning, preheat the oven to 400 degrees *as soon as you get up*. Take the French toast casserole out of the fridge. It helps to bring it to room temperature before you bake it *if you have time*. Sprinkle your French toast with a cinnamon mixture of 2 teaspoons of cinnamon and 2 tablespoons sugar.
5. Bake uncovered 30 minutes or more until golden brown and bubbly hot. Serve with a drizzle of agave syrup or honey.

Servings: 6

Nutrition Facts: Serving size: ⅙ of a recipe (7 ounces), Amount Per Serving: Calories 243, Total Fat 5g, Saturated Fat 1g, Cholesterol 106mg, Sodium 393mg, Potassium 325mg, Total Carbohydrates 38g, Fiber 5.23g, Sugar 16g, Protein 14g

Food Group Servings: 2 grain, 1protein egg group, 1 fruit

Health Coach Tips:
- Take the French toast out of the fridge as soon as you get up in the morning. It helps to bring it to room temperature before you bake it if you have time – otherwise it can take longer than 30 minutes to bake.
- Add chopped pecans or walnuts for more protein, fiber and flavor.

Pumpkin Waffles

Make a batch of these on the weekends, wrap extras well and put them in the freezer. On busy mornings, just pop them in the toaster for a quick breakfast.

1 ½ cups all-purpose flour
1 cup whole wheat flour
2 ½ teaspoons baking powder
1 teaspoon baking soda
½ teaspoon salt
2 teaspoons cinnamon
1 ½ teaspoons pumpkin pie spice

1 cup milk
1 cup shaken buttermilk
1 ¼ cups canned pumpkin
4 tablespoons Smart Balance or Earth Balance
⅓ cup brown sugar
4 large eggs, beaten

1. Sift together flours, brown sugar, baking powder, baking soda, salt, and spices.
2. In another bowl, whisk eggs in a large bowl until blended, then whisk in milk, buttermilk, and pumpkin until smooth. Whisk in dry ingredients just until smooth. Cook in waffle iron with cooking spray.

Servings: 12 (Yield: ½ cup batter).

Nutrition Facts: Serving size: $\frac{1}{12}$ of recipe (4.3 ounces) 1 waffle. Amount Per Serving: Calories 183, Total Fat 4g, Saturated Fat 1g, Cholesterol 72mg, Sodium 447mg, Potassium 206mg, Total Carbohydrates 30, Fiber 3g, Sugar 9g, Protein 7g

Food Group Servings: 2 grains, ½ vegetable

Health Coach Tips:
♥ Pumpkin is high in vitamin A from beta-carotene, which helps with vision, growth, and repair of body tissues and is an antioxidant that helps strengthen resistance to infection.
♥ Use a teaspoon of buttery spread on your cooked waffle with a drizzle of real maple syrup.

Quinoa Cinnamon Oatmeal

Combined with quinoa, this oatmeal proves you with one of the best sources of protein. Quinoa is gluten free, has a low glycemic index, and provides all of the eight essential amino acids our bodies need. Be creative and add your own ideas: chopped apples, blueberries, chopped walnuts, almonds or pecans. This large batch gives you enough to save for the next day.

1 cup quinoa

1 cup oats

4 cups water

¼ teaspoon salt

2 tablespoons brown sugar

1 teaspoon lemon juice

1 teaspoon vanilla

½ teaspoon cinnamon

¾ cup raisins

1. In a large saucepan combine oats, quinoa, water, salt, brown sugar and raisins.
2. Bring to a boil, then reduce heat and simmer for about 15 minutes or until all liquid is absorbed.
3. Add lemon juice, cinnamon and vanilla, stir and cover. Let stand for 5 minutes.
4. Serve with a splash of warm milk and teaspoon of brown sugar if desired.

Servings: 6

Nutrition Facts: Serving size: 1 cup. Serving size: ⅙ of a recipe (8 ounces), Amount Per Serving: Calories 230, Total Fat 2g, Saturated Fat 0.28g, Cholesterol 0mg, Sodium 107mg, Potassium 379mg, Total Carbohydrates 49g, Fiber 4g, Sugar 17g, Protein 6g

Food Group Servings: 2 servings of grain

Health Coach Tip:
♥ There are many ways to make oatmeal with or without the quinoa. Make it more filling and power packed with nutrition by adding flax meal, wheat germ, chopped nuts, chopped figs, dates, prunes or other dried or fresh fruit. Adding these healthy toppings will help to keep you full much longer.

Strawberry Whole Wheat Breakfast Crepes

A delicious, healthy and gourmet breakfast with a lot less sugar than the kind you get in restaurants. We make these for special Sunday breakfasts with family.

3 eggs	2 cups strawberries, sliced
1 egg white	4 tablespoons strawberry jam
¾ cup whole wheat flour	½ cup fat-free yogurt, vanilla
2 tablespoons sugar	1 cup 1% milk
½ teaspoon salt	2 tablespoons flax meal
8 tablespoons cream cheese (low-fat)	Cooking spray or buttery spread

1. Using 3 whole eggs and one egg white, mix eggs with a beater on high for at least 2 minutes.
2. Add milk and mix on high for one minute more. Gradually add flour and flax, mixing on low. Add sugar and salt, mixing on low until mixture is smooth.
3. **To make your syrup:** Add washed and sliced strawberries to a small saucepan with strawberry jam and heat until thin, about 5 minutes.
4. **Filling for crepes:** mix the cream cheese with yogurt until light and fluffy.
5. Heat a nonstick crepe pan or skillet, spray with cooking spray, or melt ½ teaspoon butter or buttery spread in pan.
6. Pour a small ladle of batter to pan, spreading the batter thin and evenly over the surface. When crepe has cooked enough so that edges will lift, flip crepe and cook briefly on the other side.
7. Make the crepes ahead and keep warm in the oven on a cookie sheet.
8. Fill each crepe with a couple of tablespoons of filling. Top with homemade strawberry syrup.

Servings: 5 (2 crepes each)

Nutrition Facts: Serving size: ⅕ of a recipe (10 ounces), Amount Per Serving: Calories 275, Total Fat 5, Saturated Fat 2g, Cholesterol 135mg, Sodium 461mg, Potassium 381mg, Total Carbohydrates 41g, Fiber 2g, Sugar 11g, Protein 16g

Food Group Servings: 1 grain, ½ fruit, 1 dairy, 1 protein egg group

Health Coach Tips:
- ♥ You get to choose the amount of fat and cholesterol in these crepes. Use egg whites or whole eggs for the batter and low-fat cream cheese and fat-free yogurt for the filling to keep the fat grams down.

Whole Wheat Coffee Cake

This special treat is only to be savored with something to balance your blood sugar, such as scrambled eggs, nuts or yogurt. It makes a great brunch side dish.

2 cups whole wheat flour	¼ teaspoon salt
1 ¼ cups all-purpose flour	1 ½ cup granulated sugar
¾ cup packed brown sugar	10 tablespoons buttery spread
½ cup walnuts, finely chopped	¾ cup egg substitute
1 teaspoon ground cinnamon	1 teaspoon vanilla extract
2 teaspoons baking soda	1 ½ cups buttermilk, 1%
1 teaspoon baking powder	Cooking spray

1. Preheat oven to 350 degrees. Coat a Bundt Pan or 10" round pan with cooking spray.
2. Combine brown sugar, walnuts, and cinnamon in a small bowl. Set aside.
3. Lightly spoon flour into dry measuring cups and if you have one, put a metal strainer over a large bowl to combine the flour, baking soda, baking powder, and salt. Sift into bowl and stir with a whisk.
4. In a large mixing bowl, combine sugar and buttery spread with a mixer on medium speed until well combined, 2 or 3 minutes. Add egg substitute, beat 3 minutes more, and add vanilla.
5. Add flour mixture and buttermilk alternately to sugar mixture, beginning and ending with flour mixture, beating well and scraping sides of bowl after each addition. Spoon half of batter into a 10-inch Bundt pan. Sprinkle half of brown sugar mixture evenly over batter; spoon remaining half of batter into pan. Top with remaining brown sugar mixture.
6. Bake at 350 degrees for 55 minutes or until a wooden toothpick inserted comes out clean. Cool in pan 10 minutes on a wire rack; remove from pan. Cool completely on wire rack.

Servings: 16

Nutrition Facts: Serving size: ¹⁄₁₆ of a recipe (3.6 ounces), Amount Per Serving: Calories 301, Total Fat 9g, Saturated Fat 2g, Cholesterol 1mg, Sodium 329mg, Potassium 135mg, Total Carbohydrates 50g, Fiber 1g, Sugar 30g, Protein 5g

Food Group Servings: 2 grain, 2 fat

Health Coach Tip:
♥ We all need a little treat now and then to help us keep on our healthy path. Slice into 16 servings so you keep your portion size real. You know it is fresh when you make it yourself.

Whole Wheat Pumpkin Muffins

Spread with light cream cheese and eat with an apple and a glass of low fat or almond milk for a quick breakfast you can take with you.

1 cup all-purpose flour	⅛ teaspoon salt
¾ cup whole wheat flour	1 egg beaten
3 tablespoons sugar	¾ cup skim milk
2 teaspoons baking powder	2 tablespoons Smart Balance
1 teaspoon pumpkin pie spice	½ cup canned pumpkin
¼ teaspoon baking soda	

1. Preheat oven to 375 degrees.
2. Spray muffin pan and or paper liners with nonstick spray.
3. In a large mixing bowl, stir together the all-purpose flour, whole wheat flour, sugar, baking powder, pumpkin pie spice, baking soda and salt. Make a well in the center.
4. In a small mixing bowl, stir together egg, milk and butter or margarine. Stir in the pumpkin. Add egg mixture all at once to dry mixture. Using a fork, stir just until moistened; batter should be lumpy.
5. Spoon batter into prepared muffin cups, filling ⅔ full. Bake in a 375 degree oven for 18 to 20 minutes or until top springs back or toothpick comes out clean.

Servings: 8

Nutrition Facts: Serving size: ⅛ of a recipe (2.9 ounces), Amount Per Serving: Calories 153, Total Fat 2g, Saturated Fat 0.64g, Cholesterol 27 mg, Sodium 274mg, Potassium 107mg, Total Carbohydrates 29g, Fiber 1g, Sugar 7g, Protein 5g

Food Group Servings: 1 grain

Health Coach Tip:
- Adding ¼ cup walnuts or pecans is a great way to add in those heart healthy nuts and added protein and fiber.
- Look for organic whole grain flours such as King Arthur, Bob's Red Mill.
- Or look for ancient grains or a milled blend of 30% each amaranth, millet, and sorghum flours, plus 10% quinoa flour—100% whole grain, with all the bran and germ. Adds protein and amino acids, along with fiber, vitamins, and minerals, to bread, muffins, cookies, and more.

Lunches You Will Love

~

Apple Walnut Salad

Serve this with a cup of your favorite soup for an easy and healthy lunch.

2 apples, diced	½ cup fat-free plain yogurt
¼ cup golden raisins	1 teaspoon lemon juice
¼ cup walnuts, roughly chopped	1 teaspoon honey

1. Wash and dice apple, leaving the peel on. Sprinkle with lemon juice to keep from turning brown.
2. Toss apples with remaining ingredients.

Servings: 3

Nutrition Facts: Serving size: ⅓ of a recipe (5.6 ounces), Amount Per Serving: Calories 181, Total Fat 3g, Saturated Fat 1g, Cholesterol 2mg, Sodium 31mg, Potassium 330mg, Total Carbohydrates 29g, Fiber 4g, Sugar 22g, Protein 4g

Food Group Servings: 1 fruit, 1 dairy, 1 fat

Health Coach Tip:
- ♥ This also makes a very nutritious snack in a ½ cup serving. Apples are known for their soluble fiber that helps lower cholesterol and aids in evening out blood sugar levels. Instead of just eating plain fruit for a snack, the added protein and healthy fat helps you feel full longer.

Asian Noodle Salad

This flavorful recipe comes from Professor and Chef Clare Dendinger, MA, CFCS, Professor and Chef, one of my teachers who helped me to learn about nutritious cooking. Her enthusiasm inspired me to be more creative in my own meals.

6 ounces whole wheat spaghetti	3 Tablespoons sesame seeds, toasted
1 ½ Teaspoons sesame oil, divided	¼ cup rice-wine vinegar
8 ounces asparagus spears	1 tablespoon honey
8 ounces snow peas	½ tablespoon sesame oil
Salt and pepper to taste	1 teaspoon Chinese five spice
6 green onions (scallions), sliced	1 clove garlic, minced
1 large red bell pepper seeded and sliced	

1. Snap the fibrous ends off the asparagus and cut the stalk sharply on the diagonal into 2" pieces. Set aside with washed snow peas.
2. Cook the noodles in 4 quarts of boiling water until done, al dente, 6 to 8 minutes.
3. During the last two minutes of cooking the pasta, add the asparagus, and then the last minute add the snow peas. Drain all in colander, rinse with cold water, and drain well. Transfer to a large mixing bowl and toss with 1 Teaspoon sesame oil.
4. To prepare the dressing: mash the garlic and half the sesame seeds and put into an attractive serving bowl. Add the vinegar, honey, remaining ½ Teaspoon sesame oil and seasonings; whisk until blended. Correct the seasoning at the time.
5. Add the noodles, asparagus, snow peas, bell pepper, scallion whites, and half of the scallion greens to the dressing and toss to mix.
6. Sprinkle the remaining sesame seeds and scallion greens on top to serve.

Servings: 6

Nutrition Facts: Serving size: ⅙ of a recipe (5.6 ounces), Amount Per Serving: Calories 127, Total Fat 5g, Saturated Fat 0.7g, Cholesterol 0mg, Sodium 8mg, Potassium 336.22mg, Total Carbohydrates 22.23g, Fiber 4g, Sugar 6g, Protein 5g

Food group servings: 1 Vegetable, 1 grain, 1 fat

Health Coach Tips:
- ♥ To add more protein, toss your salad with a couple of tablespoons of peanuts or a cup of diced tofu or cooked chicken.
- ♥ Bell peppers are low in calories, and all colors are rich in fiber and vitamins A & C.

Notice this recipe is low in sodium because we don't use soy sauce.

Best Chicken Salad

The key to good chicken salad is to keep it simple. Roast or poach your chicken with a little salt and pepper and drizzle of olive oil. Everyone loves this lower fat chicken salad recipe.

3 boneless skinless chicken breasts

4 tablespoons fat free or light mayonnaise

1 teaspoon lemon juice

2 tablespoons plain fat-free yogurt

¾ cup celery, chopped

2 teaspoons olive oil

Salt and pepper to taste

1. Preheat oven to 350 degrees.
2. Salt and pepper chicken breast and lightly rub with olive oil. Place on a baking sheet and roast for 20 minutes or until no longer pink. You can also poach your chicken in a pan of chicken broth on the stove for 12-20 minutes or until done.
3. Cool chicken to room temperature. Dice chicken and put in a mixing bowl.
4. Mix remaining ingredients and serve as a sandwich or salad.

Servings: 8

Nutrition Facts: Serving size: ⅛ of a recipe (4 ounces), Amount Per Serving: Calories 150, Total Fat 6, Saturated Fat 1g, Cholesterol 54mg, Sodium 152mg, Potassium 259mg, Total Carbohydrates 2g, Fiber <1g, Sugar <1g, Protein 20g

Food Group Servings: 1 Meat, 1 fat

Health Coach Tips:

♥ When you order chicken salad in a restaurant, you have no idea how much full fat mayonnaise they use, so you have no idea of the calories you are eating. There are 1,440 calories in one cup of regular mayonnaise and 160 grams of fat! Best food light only has 1 gram of fat per tablespoon instead of 10 grams for regular and it takes great.

♥ Chicken salad on a bed of lettuce with other sliced veggies makes a great dinner on a hot day, then use extra for lunch box sandwiches.

♥ When cooked without the skin chicken is a good low-fat (*only 3 grams per 3 ounces*) source of protein and several B vitamins including vitamin B6, B12 and niacin which are important for healthy immune function.

Harvest Salad

I made this salad for each group when I taught the Diabetes Prevention Program at our local health clinic. It was a favorite recipe because of the sweet and savory contrast. I still make it often and use the low-fat salad dressing recipe for many salads.

3 heads of romaine lettuce, shredded
2 apples, diced with peels on
2 pears, dices with peels on
¼ cup golden raisins
2 tablespoons sunflower seeds
1 yellow bell pepper, chopped
2 carrots, peeled and grated
½ purple onion, thinly sliced

Salad Dressing:
1 tablespoon Extra-virgin olive oil
3 tablespoons apple cider vinegar
1 tablespoon honey
¼ cup water
Salt and pepper to taste

1. Wash, dry and shred the lettuce.
2. Dice the apples, pears and bell pepper, and add to lettuce in a large bowl.
3. Thinly slice red onion and add to the salad with raisins and sunflower seeds.
4. Mix all salad dressing ingredients in a jar with a lid and shake. Toss the salad just before serving.

Servings: 4

Nutrition Facts: Serving size: ¼ of a recipe, (1 ½ cups), Amount Per Serving: Calories 230, Total Fat 6, Saturated Fat <1g, Cholesterol 0mg, Sodium 170mg, Total Carbohydrates 42g, Fiber 7g, Sugar 30g, Protein 4g

Food Group Servings: 2 Fruit, 1 ½ vegetable

Health Coach Tip: Sunflower seeds provide an array of protective nutrients. They are high in vitamin E, an essential vitamin with antioxidant and anti-inflammatory effects that help protect the heart and reduce the risk of diabetic complications. Additionally, sunflower seeds can help lower cholesterol.

Blue Cheese, Walnut & Berry Salad

Compared to other nuts, walnuts provide the most omega-3 fats. If you are not a fan of blue cheese, this is delicious with feta cheese. It is filling enough for a main meal served with a multigrain roll or cup of soup.

2 cups baby spinach, washed and chopped
1 cup strawberries, sliced
½ cup fresh raspberries
¼ cup crumbled blue cheese or feta
½ cup walnuts, roughly chopped
2 cups romaine lettuce, shredded

Salad Dressing:
2 tablespoons olive oil
3 tablespoons red wine vinegar
1 teaspoon sugar or honey
½ cup fresh blackberries
Salt and pepper to taste

1. To make salad dressing: Place a few berries in the blender with the oil, vinegar, sugar or honey and a little salt and pepper and whirl until mixed.
2. Toss remaining ingredients, except cheese in a large bowl with dressing. Serve on individual salad plates topped with a sprinkle of the blue cheese.

Servings: 4

Nutrition Facts: Serving size: ¼ of a recipe (11.4 ounces), Amount Per Serving: Calories 211, Total Fat 14g, Saturated Fat 3g, Cholesterol 5mg, Sodium 128mg, Potassium 382g, Total Carbohydrates 12, Fiber 4g, Sugar 6g, Protein 4g

Food Group Servings: 1 Fruit, 1 vegetable, 1 fat

Health Coach Tips:
- ♥ Walnuts are a delicious and healthy way to get omega-3 fats, which we all need to balance with omega 6 fats. Eaten in proper portions walnuts are helpful for people with diabetes and in preventing diabetes and heart disease as they help reduce insulin resistance and excess body weight.
- ♥ The good amounts of omega-3 fats also help prevent blood clotting, reduce inflammation and lower triglyceride levels in the blood. Walnuts also supply protein and soluble fiber-a combination of nutrients that helps to satisfy hunger, lower cholesterol and smooth out blood sugar fluctuations.

Greek Pasta Salad

Pasta is not to be avoided. It has a low glycemic index and does not spike blood sugar. The key is to eat **proper portions**-*that means less pasta pumped up with lots of vegetables*! This is a filling salad rich with vegetables. Make it ahead of time so the pasta can absorb all the flavors, then toss again before serving.

3 cups diced tomatoes	¾ cup sliced red onions
⅓ cup sliced black olives	⅓ cup halved green olives
5 ounces crumbled feta cheese	1 cup bell pepper, chopped
One (12) ounce bag pasta- *I like Barilla Plus*	One (15 ounce) can garbanzo beans, drained
1 cup marinated mushrooms, drained	1 jar marinated artichoke hearts, drained
1 cup cucumbers peeled, cut into ¼ -inch slices	1 Tablespoon dried oregano

Dressing:

¼ cup olive oil	3 tablespoons lemon juice
2 Tablespoons water	3 tablespoons balsamic vinegar
2 Teaspoons crushed garlic	

1. For optimal nutrition, use wholegrain or Barilla Pasta Plus which is made from nutritious things such as chickpeas and egg whites. For fun you can mix two types such as Rotini and Farfalle (bowties).
2. Cook pasta according to directions on package, drain and place in serving bowl. Add all chopped vegetables, feta cheese, and oregano.
3. Mix dressing ingredients together, pour over salad and toss. Chill in refrigerator for at least an hour before serving to allow flavors to come together. Sprinkle more feta cheese over the top to serve. Add 1 cup of cherry tomatoes and pitted Kalamata olives, to kick up the flavor.

Servings: 8.Nutrition Facts: Serving size: ⅛ of a recipe (7.8 ounces), Amount Per Serving: Calories 224, Total Fat 13g, Saturated Fat 4g, Cholesterol 16mg, Sodium 407mg, Potassium 448mg, Total Carbohydrates 23g, Fiber 6g, Sugar 5g, Protein 7g

Food Group Servings: 2 Vegetable, 1 grain, 2 fat

Health Coach Tip:
♥ Before serving, add a splash of oil and vinegar or water if salad is too dry. Garbanzo beans add protein. Beans are legumes and are packed with vitamins and minerals and are rich in fiber. Eating 1 ½ cups of various kinds of beans per week can help reduce the risk of heart disease and certain cancers and are an excellent replacement for meat.

Grilled Lime Fajitas

This is a quick yet flavorful recipe for lunch or dinner. You can also make fajitas with chicken or fish to reduce saturated fat.

12 flour or whole wheat tortillas
¼ cup cilantro
1 tablespoon chili powder
3 cloves garlic, minced
2 red bell pepper, thinly sliced
¾ pound flank steak
2 yellow bell peppers seeded and sliced thin

¼ cup lime juice
¼ cup vinegar
1 tablespoon pepper
2 green bell peppers, seeded and sliced thin
1 red onion, sliced thin
¼ cup olive oil for marinade (poured off)

1. Mix together lime juice, cilantro, vinegar, oil, garlic, and spices. Marinate meat in mixture overnight.
2. Pour off marinade and grill bell peppers, onions, and meat. To make your fajitas indoors, heat a lightly oiled grill pan or heavy skillet over medium heat and cook the steak until seared on both sides, about 5 minutes for medium rare and 10 minutes for medium well done. Grill the vegetables the last few minutes with your meat. Slice meat in thin strips against the grain.
3. Warm your tortillas without oil in a skillet or in the oven or on the grill in foil. Serve the meat and vegetables on a platter with tortillas, along with toppings such as salsa, light sour cream or nonfat plain yogurt, avocado, sliced green onions and lime slices.

Servings: 6.

Nutrition Facts: Serving size: ⅙ of a recipe (10.7 ounces), Amount Per Serving: Calories 307, Total Fat 11g, Saturated Fat 3g, Cholesterol 23mg, Sodium 56mg, Potassium 631mg, Total Carbohydrates 37g, Fiber 6g, Sugar 3g, Protein 17g

Food Group Servings: 1 Vegetable, 2 grains, 1 meat, 1 fat

Health Coach Tip:
♥ **Onions** contain the mineral chromium which plays a crucial role for people with diabetes by enhancing insulin's ability to lower blood sugar levels. Like **garlic,** onions appear to promote heart health by lowering blood cholesterol levels and reduce blood clotting. Onions also contain phytonutrients that fight inflammation and improve blood vessel health.

Asian Cabbage Chicken Salad

A delicious and nutrious lunch. To make this vegetarian, simply leave out the chicken.

5 cups Napa or green cabbage, shredded
1 cup carrots, grated
1 cup snow peas
½ cup red bell pepper, seeded and diced
2 green onions, sliced
2 cucumbers, sliced ¼-inch thin
6 green onion, sliced
4 chicken breasts, boned and skinned
1 Tablespoon Mrs. Dash no salt seasoning

2 tablespoons olive oil, extra-virgin, divided
¼ cup rice-wine vinegar
1 teaspoon garlic powder
1 tablespoon peanut butter
¼ cup peanuts
1 tablespoon brown sugar
5 tablespoons soy sauce, low-sodium
¼ cup water

1. Wash and pat dry chicken breasts and place in a baking dish prepared with cooking spray. Sprinkle chicken with Mrs. Dash no salt seasoning and drizzle chicken with 1 tablespoon olive oil. Roast at 350 degrees until done, about 15-20 minutes or until juices run clear. Cool then thinly slice the chicken.
2. **To make salad dressing**: whisk 1 tablespoon of the olive oil, low-sodium soy sauce, vinegar, garlic powder, peanut butter, brown sugar and ¼ cup water.
3. Wash, slice or dice the vegetables: cabbage, carrots, green onions, snow peas (or sugar snap peas), cucumber, and place in a large bowl. Toss with salad dressing just before serving then top with sliced chicken, green onions and peanuts.

6 servings: ⅙ of the recipe about 2 cups.

Nutrition facts per serving: 316 calories, fat 11g, cholesterol 91mg, sodium 649mg, carbohydrates 21g, fiber 5g, sugar 9g, protein 42g

Food Group Servings: 1 meat, 2 vegetables, 1 fat

Health Coach Tips:
♥ Researchers have found that eating leafy green vegetables such as cabbage may reduce the risk of developing type 2 diabetes. Savoy and bok choy reduce the risk of certain cancers and heart disease. Cabbage offers fiber to help slow blood sugar's rise during a meal. All types of cabbage are low in calories and high in nutrition. Chinese or Napa cabbage works great in this salad. Purple cabbage adds color.

Hearty Chicken Tortilla Soup

If you have pre-cooked chicken, you can add that with the broth to save time. *Many of these ingredients are optional.* Use any type of beans and other vegetables you have such as celery, zucchini and carrots for this easy recipe.

1 tablespoon olive oil

2 teaspoons dried oregano

4 tablespoons lime juice

One (15) oz can black beans, drained

4 chicken breasts, boned and skinned

1 avocado, cut into ½ -inch dice

4 large garlic cloves, minced

One 28-ounce can diced tomatoes

10 corn tortillas (6 inches)

One 15-ounce can pinto beans, drained

½ cup chopped fresh cilantro

One 28-ounce can crushed tomatoes

4 teaspoons chili powder

One 16-ounce package frozen corn

Two 4-ounce can green chilies, chopped

One 32-ounce can chicken broth with no msg

2 medium onions, finely chopped

1. Preheat oven to 325 degrees. Lay corn tortillas on a cookie sheet and spray with cooking spray. Bake in oven for about 10 minutes or until lightly crisp. Save for later.
2. Heat oil in large Dutch oven or soup pan over medium heat.
3. Sauté onions about 3 minutes until soft. Add chicken and season with garlic, chili powder, and oregano. Brown slightly for a couple of minutes. Add tomatoes, broth, corn, chilies, and beans and bring to a simmer.
4. Reduce heat and cook on low for 20 minutes until the flavors come together.
5. To serve, layer sliced tortillas in bottom of a bowl, ladle in soup. Garnish with cilantro and a Tablespoon of avocado and other optional ingredients such light sour cream or 2 Tablespoons shredded jack cheese. (*Just remember to add the extra fat to your daily total*)

Servings: 12. **Nutrition Facts**: Serving size: ¹⁄₁₂ of a recipe (about 2 cups), Amount Per Serving: Calories 270, Total Fat 6g, Saturated Fat <1g, Cholesterol 46g, Sodium 650mg, Potassium 858mg, Total Carbohydrates 32g, Fiber 7g, Sugar 5, Protein 25g

Food Group Servings: 2 Vegetable, 2 meat/bean, 1 grain

Health Coach Tip: Vegetarians can easily make this dish by substituting the chicken broth and chicken for the vegetable broth and diced tofu. The flavors are still spicy and delicious.

Light & Fluffy Egg Salad Sandwich

The key to great egg salad is to cook the eggs properly, then grate the hardboiled eggs with a cheese grater. After gently boiling the eggs, rinse in cold water to help the shell peel off easily.

4 eggs	2 egg whites
1 teaspoon lemon juice	3 teaspoons fat free mayonnaise
Salt and pepper to taste	1 teaspoon Dijon style mustard
6 slices 100% whole grain bread	3 teaspoons mayonnaise or fat-free Greek yogurt

1. Bring eggs to a boil in a medium size saucepan on the stove, then turn off the heat, cover and let stand for 12 minutes. Immediately take them out of the pan and put in a bowl, then under cold running water. Turn off the water and let them cool.
2. In a mixing bowl, mix both types of mayonnaise or yogurt, lemon juice and mustard.
3. Peel shell off eggs, rinse in water to make sure you get all the shells off. Pat dry with a paper towel. Slice two of the eggs in half and discard two of the yolks.
4. Grate all the eggs and egg whites over a mixing bowl with a cheese grater.
5. Gently combine the grated eggs with remaining ingredients to mix. Spread on two slices of the freshest whole-grain bread.

Servings: 3. **Nutrition Facts**: Serving size: ⅓ of a recipe (5.9 ounces), Amount Per Serving: Calories 29, Total Fat 12g, Saturated Fat 3g, Cholesterol 322mg, Sodium 485mg, Potassium 275mg, Total Carbohydrates 26g, Fiber 4g, Sugar 5g, Protein 19.g

Food Group Servings: 2 Grains, 2 eggs, 1 fat

Health Coach Tips:
- ♥ If you love egg salad but want to reduce the cholesterol even more, discard more egg yolks and add ground garbanzo beans and substitute fat-free yogurt for the mayonnaise.
- ♥ Save time by making lunches the night before. Want a way to get your kids to switch to whole grain bread? Start by making sandwiches with 1 slice wheat and 1 slice of buttermilk bread. Call them half-and-half sandwiches. They will love it.
- ♥ For years eggs have been given some negative press, but as it turns out research indicates they can be a healthy addition to any meal plan. Eggs offer 13 essential vitamins and minerals, high quality protein, healthy unsaturated fats and are low in calories. Eating eggs for breakfast controls hunger and blood sugar levels. For those with a history of heart disease the American Heart Association recommends limiting eggs to 3 per week.

Light n' Creamy Pumpkin Soup

This soup is low in calories, yet packed with nutrition. While traditional pumpkin soup is made with cream, substitute fat-free or low-fat milk and you will save on calories and fat without sacrificing flavor.

2 teaspoons healthy buttery spread
¾ teaspoon sage
¼ teaspoon nutmeg
1 tablespoon tomato paste
1 cup chopped peeled apple
3 cups cubed peeled fresh pumpkin or canned

1 cup chopped onion
½ teaspoon curry powder
3 tablespoons all-purpose flour
¼ teaspoon salt
½ cup 1% milk or fat-free plain yogurt
Three 10.5-ounce cans low-sodium, chicken broth

1. Melt buttery spread in a Dutch oven over medium heat. Add onion, sauté for 3 minutes. Add sage, curry, and nutmeg. Cook for 30 seconds.
2. Stir in flour; cook 30 seconds. Add broth, tomato paste, and salt, stirring well with a whisk. Stir in pumpkin and apple. Bring to a boil. Cover, reduce heat and simmer 25 minutes or until pumpkin is tender, stir occasionally. (For canned pumpkin cooking time is 10 min).
3. Remove from heat and cool slightly.
4. Place mixture in a blender or food processor or use an emersion blender until smooth.
5. Return mixture to Dutch oven; add milk. Cook until thoroughly heated.

Servings: 5. **Nutrition Facts**: Serving size: ⅕ of a recipe (2 cups) Amount Per Serving: Calories 181 Total Fat 4g, Saturated Fat 0g, Cholesterol 1mg, Sodium 589mg, Potassium 753mg, Total Carbohydrates 28g, Fiber 5g, Sugar 16, Protein 9g

Food Group Servings: 1 Vegetable, 1, fat

Health Coach Tips:
- ♥ Remember that you can healthfully, make any of the cream soups you love from cream of broccoli to lobster bisque by substituting milk or evaporated milk mixed with a little flour or cornstarch. *Why should we leave out the heavy cream?* Because every cup of heavy cream contains 821 calories, 88 grams of fat and 326 mg of cholesterol.
- ♥ **Pumpkin** is loaded with fiber, vitamins and minerals. The average American doesn't get enough of the recommended 20-35 grams of daily fiber. One cup of pumpkin puree provides you with 7.1 grams of fiber. A one cup serving also supplies 3.4 grams

of iron, a mineral that helps you from getting sick by supporting a strong immune system, plus 1906 micrograms of vitamin A which keeps your eyes, bones and teeth healthy. Pumpkin also provides vitamin E and reduces inflammation which helps prevent cancer, heart disease, Type 2 diabetes and arthritis. Wow, what a powerhouse of nutrients!

Minestrone Soup

Add any vegetables you have to this soup, making it with or without beef. You can make this vegetarian by leaving out the beef and using vegetable broth and wine. Either way this recipe is easy, nutritious, and filling. It freezes well, so make a big batch for lunches and dinners.

3 cups water
¼ teaspoon pepper
1 cup water
2 tablespoons flour
½ cup Parmesan cheese, grated
1 cup spinach or kale stripped off stock, chopped
1 cup shell shaped pasta, small
One 15-ounce can diced tomatoes

1 onion chopped
1 tablespoon olive oil
1 zucchini thinly sliced
2 carrots sliced
½ pound beef sirloin
One 16-ounce can garbanzo beans
1 ½ teaspoons Italian seasoning
1 cup shell shaped pasta, small

1 teaspoon salt
2 cloves garlic minced
2 cups chopped cabbage
½ cup red wine
2 cups chicken broth or water
1 cup celery with leaves chopped
2 tablespoons minced parsley
½ pound beef sirloin

1. You can make this soup without meat. If you want to use beef, choose a lean cut and trim all the visible fat off. Cut into 1" cubes. Put olive oil in a heavy soup pot and add onion, stir lightly until translucent. Add beef to brown meat for a few minutes. Add garlic and wine.
2. Combine in soup pot water, salt, pepper, Italian seasoning, parsley, tomatoes, celery, zucchini, cabbage, spinach, and carrots. Drain and rinse garbanzo and other beans, add to soup and stir all. Bring to a boil then add pasta, turning heat to simmer for 10 to 20 minutes or until all the vegetables are done and the flavors deepen. Serve with a sprinkle of parmesan cheese.

Servings: 10

Nutrition Facts: Serving size: (15 ounces about 2 cups), Amount Per Serving: Calories 250, Total Fat 6g, Saturated Fat 2g, Cholesterol 23mg, Sodium 820 mg, Potassium 682mg, Total Carbohydrates 31g, Fiber 6g, Sugar 5g, Protein 16g

Food Group Servings: 2 Vegetable, ½ serving grain, 1 meat, 2 fat

Health Coach Tip:
♥ This minestrone can be made in the slow cooker or on the stove. In the slow cooker, wait to add the pasta and cabbage the last 30 minutes to avoid over cooking. You can always add more vegetables for added nutrition.

Polenta Pizza

You make this simple pizza with a baked polenta crust and can top it with your favorites: mushrooms, onions, turkey sausage, olives-*make it your way. It is easy and delicious.*

1 Tablespoon olive oil
1 cup polenta (or cornmeal)
¼ cup freshly grated Parmesan cheese
1 cup sliced mushrooms

1 fresh tomato, diced
½ red onion, sliced thin
4 ounces Mozzarella cheese, shredded
2 Tablespoons fresh basil, chopped

1. Pre-heat oven to 400 degrees. Spray a 9-inch pie plate.
2. In a medium saucepan, bring 2 ¼ cups water to a boil. Whisking constantly, slowly add your polenta or cornmeal. Reduce heat to low and cook, stirring, until the polenta starts to pull away from the side of the pan, 4 to 5 minutes. Stir in the parmesan, ½ teaspoon salt, and ¼ Teaspoon pepper. Using a spoon spread the polenta over the bottom and up the sides of the prepared pan.
3. In a bowl, combine the mushrooms, onions, tomatoes, mozzarella cheese, the remaining Tablespoon of oil, and ¼ Teaspoon each of salt and pepper. Spoon the mixture over the polenta and bake until the polenta is crisp around the edges, about 25 to 30 minutes. Sprinkle with chopped basil and serve.

Servings: 4

Nutrition Facts: Serving size: ¼ of a recipe (5.1 ounces), Amount Per Serving: Calories 291, Calories From Fat 92.46, Total Fat 11g, Saturated Fat 5g, Cholesterol 24mg, Sodium 277mg, Potassium 231.7mg, Total Carbohydrates 35.62g, Fiber 2g, Sugar 2g, Protein 13g

Food Group Servings: 1 Vegetable, 1 grain, 1 fat

Health Coach Tip:
♥   To make a crispier crust, put it in the oven and bake for 5 minutes before you add the toppings.

Vegetarian Fried Rice

Using brown rice instead of white makes this a very nutritious dish. Make the brown rice ahead of time so you can whip this up for a very quick meal.

3 cups cooked brown rice
1 teaspoon canola oil
½ cup sliced fresh mushrooms
½ cup shredded carrot
½ cup chopped green bell pepper
¼ teaspoon ginger

1 clove garlic minced
2 tablespoons light soy sauce or Bragg
   Liquid Aminos
2 eggs beaten
⅛ teaspoon pepper
¾ cup frozen peas, thawed

1. While rice is cooking, spray large nonstick skillet or wok with nonstick cooking spray, add 1 Teaspoon of canola oil and heat over medium heat until hot. Add mushrooms, carrot, onions, bell pepper, ginger, and garlic; cook and stir one minute.
2. Reduce heat to low. Stir in rice and soy sauce; cook 2 minutes stirring occasionally.
3. Push rice mixture to side of skillet, add eggs, and pepper to the other side. Cook over low heat for 2 minutes to come together, then flip and lightly brown the other side. Slice the eggs up into thin ribbons.
4. Add peas to rice and egg mixture; stir gently to combine. Season with pepper and cook until thoroughly heated. If desired, serve with additional soy sauce.

Servings: 6

Nutrition Facts: Serving size: ⅙ of a recipe (5.6 ounces), Amount Per Serving: Calories 164, Total Fat 3g, Saturated Fat 0.7g, Cholesterol 70mg, Sodium 251mg, Potassium 198mg, Total Carbohydrates 27g, Fiber 3g, Sugar 2g, Protein 6g

Food Group Servings: 1 Vegetable, 1 grain

Health Coach Tips:
- To quickly thaw peas, place in a colander or strainer, and rinse with warm water until thawed.
- If you want to make a main dish out of this, add cooked diced ham, pork or bacon to the onion and bell pepper mixture.

Fast, Fresh & Healthy Dinners

~

Barbecue Roasted Salmon

This easy, flavorful recipe will make a fish lover out of anyone. Serve with brown rice and stir fried vegetables to round out a nutritious meal.

¼ cup pineapple juice
2 tablespoons fresh lemon juice
Four (6 ounce) salmon fillets
2 tablespoons brown sugar
4 teaspoons chili powder
2 teaspoons grated lemon rind

¾ teaspoon ground cumin
½ teaspoon salt
¼ teaspoon ground cinnamon
Cooking spray
Lemon slices

1. Combine first 3 ingredients in a plastic bag, seal and marinate in refrigerator for 1 hour, turning occasionally.
2. Preheat oven to 400 degrees.
3. Remove fish from bag; discard marinade. Combine sugar and next 5 ingredients (sugar through cinnamon) in a bowl. Rub all over fish.
4. Grill on barbecue or place in a baking dish coated with cooking spray and bake in 400 degree oven for 12 minutes or until fish flakes easily with a fork. Serve with lemon slices.

Servings: 8

Nutrition Facts: Serving size: ⅛ of a recipe (4.4 ounces), Amount Per Serving: Calories 167, Total Fat 6g, Saturated Fat 1g, Cholesterol 54mg, Sodium 204mg, Potassium 543mg, Total Carbohydrates 6g, Fiber 0.62g, Sugar 4g, Protein 20g

Food Group Servings: 1 Serving = 1 Meat, 1 fat

Snapper Veracruz

This recipe makes a fish lover out of everyone.

One 15-ounce can diced tomatoes
2 medium white onions sliced into rings
1 tablespoon of extra-virgin olive oil
2 medium green bell peppers thinly sliced
1 teaspoon of salt and pepper, or to taste
2 pounds of red snapper fillets cut into 5
    ounce pieces

1 teaspoon of dried oregano
½ cup of dry white wine or water
¾ cup of chicken broth with no MSG
1 garlic clove, minced
1 tablespoon of fresh parsley
2 medium red bell pepper seeded and
    sliced

1. Spray the bottom of a 9 x 13 baking pan with cooking spray and layer with onions.
2. Arrange the Red Snapper fillets over the onions. Place the bell pepper rings over the
   Red Snapper fillets.
3. In a saucepan, combine the tomatoes, olive oil, salt, pepper, oregano, chicken broth,
   wine, and garlic. Heat to a simmer and pour over the fish. Bake for 350 degrees for
   15-20 minutes. Garnish with fresh parsley.

Serving Size: 5 oz plus 1 cup of sauce

Food Group Servings = 1 protein, 2 vegetable, 1 fat

Nutrition Facts: Serving size: 5 ounces, plus 1 cup of sauce. Amount Per Serving: Calories
230, Total Fat 4.5g, Saturated Fat 1g, Cholesterol 55mg, Sodium 370mg, Carbohydrates
13g, Fiber 3g, Sugar 7g, Protein 33g

Health Coach Tip:
♥ Serve with brown rice and a tossed green salad for a nutritious meal. Recipe can also
  be made with chicken breasts.

Salmon Patties

This recipe comes from my Aunt Dorothy and makes a quick healthy dinner. These salmon patties are also great cold in your lunch box.

2 large cans pink or red salmon
⅓ cup chopped green onions
1 egg beaten
1 egg white, slightly beaten
1 tablespoon lemon juice

¼ teaspoon salt and pepper to taste
16 each saltine crackers crushed
1 teaspoon seafood seasoning
2 tablespoons olive oil, divided

1. Drain salmon and remove skin and bones. Stir and break up salmon with a fork. Add seasonings, lemon juice, eggs, and stir. Blend in crackers. Divide in ¼ cup portions and handling lightly shape into round flat patties about ½ inch thick.
2. Heat 1 tablespoon of oil in a heavy skillet. Place patties in one skillet and brown slowly on both sides to a rich golden color. Add one more tablespoon of oil to the pan when you flip them over.

Servings: 8

Nutrition Facts: Serving size: ⅛ of a recipe (4.8 ounces), Amount Per Serving: Calories 283, Total Fat 11g, Saturated Fat 2g, Cholesterol 36mg, Sodium 511mg, Potassium 321mg, Total Carbohydrates 20g, Protein 24g

Food Group Servings = 1.5 Meat, 1 fat

Health Coach Tips:
- Using too much oil when cooking is a hidden cause of weight gain for most people. Always be aware of how much oil you add to your pan because oil or butter adds about 100 calories per tablespoon. We need fat for our health, for flavor and to help us feel full, but we tend to eat more than we realize.
- Most of the fat in Salmon comes from omega-3s, healthy polyunsaturated fatty acids. Omega-3 fish oil helps protect against heart disease and diabetes because it improves the body's ability to respond to insulin. Omega-3s may also stimulate secretion of leptin, a hormone that helps regulate food intake, body weight and metabolism.

San Francisco Cioppino

Cioppino is a fish stew originating in San Francisco and derived from the various fish soups of Italian cuisine. It is traditionally made from the catch of the day, typically a combination of crab, clams, scallops, mussels and fish. The seafood is combined with fresh tomatoes and wine. It is perfect with toasted sourdough bread on a cold night.

1 large onion, chopped

1 tablespoon of olive oil

4 cloves garlic, minced

1 green pepper chopped

One 16- ounce can tomatoes, diced

8 ounces low-sodium tomato sauce

1 or 2 Dungeness crabs cooked, cleaned
  and sectioned

2 teaspoons finely chopped parsley

1 pinch sugar

2 cups dry white wine

1 pound prawns, peeled and deveined

1 pound fish, cod, tuna, clams, mussels

One (14.5) ounce can chicken broth

2 tablespoons chopped fresh basil or 1 ½
  teaspoon dried basil

1. Heat oil in a large stockpot. Add onion, sauté until soft. Add garlic and bell pepper, cook 5 minutes. Add tomatoes, tomato sauce, broth, wine, parsley, basil, and sugar. Bring to a boil. Reduce heat and simmer, covered for 20 minutes. (The broth can be made ahead at this point and refrigerated. Reheat before adding seafood.)
2. Add crab, cover, and simmer 5 minutes. Stir in remaining seafood. Simmer 5 to 10 minutes until shrimp is pink and clams and mussels are open. (Discard those that do not open.) Be careful not to overcook seafood or it will get tough.
3. Serve with crusty French bread and a tossed green salad.

Servings: 6

Nutrition Facts: Serving size: ⅙ of a recipe (15.9 ounces), Amount Per Serving: Calories 333, Total Fat 7g, Saturated Fat 1g, Cholesterol 162mg, Sodium 729g, Potassium 878mg, Total Carbohydrates 11g, Fiber 2g, Sugar 5g, Protein 41.05g

Food Group Servings: 1 Serving = .5 Vegetable, 2 meat, 1 fats

Health Coach Tip:
- Eating at least two servings of fish each week offers multiple health benefits and is of special value to people with diabetes and heart disease, such as improving the body's handling of blood sugar and warding off diseases. Fish rich in omega3 fats include salmon, mackerel, sardines, anchovies, trout, tuna, whitefish, bass, ocean perch and halibut.

Lighter Country Rigatoni

Serve this popular classic and your guests will have no idea it is lower in fat and healthy too!

3 Italian turkey sausages
12 ounces rigatoni pasta
2 tablespoons extra-virgin olive oil
2 tablespoons crushed garlic
1 large fresh white onion, diced
3 cups broccoli florets, fresh

¼ cup chopped basil leaves
¼ cup chopped fresh parsley
2 cups canned white navy or cannellini beans
2 cups reduced sodium, fat-free chicken broth
½ cup parmesan and Romano cheese, grated

1. Bring a large pot filled with water to a rolling boil and add your pasta. Cook as directed on package. Add the broccoli for the last minute or two, then drain, reserving about 1 cup of the liquid.
2. In a large sauté pan, heat the olive oil over medium heat. When the oil is hot, sauté the onions and garlic for about 3 minutes, until golden brown being careful not to burn the garlic.
3. Add the sausage (removed from casings), basil and parsley to the onions in the pan. Break up the sausage using a wooden spoon or spatula. Cook for about 5 minutes or until the sausage is browned. Add the beans, chicken stock and bring the sauce to a boil. Reduce the heat slightly and simmer it briskly for 5-8 minutes until it starts to thicken. Stir in ¼ cup of the cheese.
4. In a large serving bowl, toss the pasta and broccoli with your sauce. Top with remaining cheese. Serve with a tossed green salad.

Servings: 8

Serving size: ⅛ of a recipe (1 cup) Amount Per Serving: Calories 340, Total Fat 11g, Saturated Fat 2g, Cholesterol 25mg, Sodium 670mg, Total Carbohydrates 45g, Fiber 5g, Sugar 3g, Protein 18g

Food Group Servings: 1 Serving = 1 Vegetable, ½ Meat, ½ Fat, ½ Beans

Health Coach Tip:
♥ You can use multi-grain pasta to add even more fiber to this well rounded meal.

Veggie & Chicken Enchilada Casserole

Layering the enchiladas into a baking dish is easier than rolling each one. These taste great and are not loaded with cheese-*saving you lots of fat and calories.*

2 Yukon Gold potatoes, cubed
1 yellow onion, peeled and chopped
½ bell pepper, chopped
½ red bell pepper seeded and chopped
1 large can enchilada sauce
½ cup light sour cream *or fat-free plain yogurt*
3 boneless chicken breasts cooked & cooled

½ teaspoon cumin
1 tablespoon canola oil
1 teaspoon chili powder
24 corn tortillas (about 6-inches)
1 teaspoon garlic powder or chopped fresh garlic
2 cups shredded Mexican-style cheese blend

1. Preheat your oven to 350 degrees. Place chicken breasts in a baking dish and drizzle with 1 teaspoon of olive oil. Sprinkle with salt, pepper, chili powder, garlic powder and roast about 30 minutes or until done. Let cool slightly, and then chop.
2. While chicken is roasting, sauté chopped onion, peppers and potatoes in 1 teaspoon of oil. Add a little water while stirring until potatoes are tender, about 15 minutes. (You can also use leftover diced potatoes for this step.)
3. Heat enchilada sauce in a saucepan. Dip 6 tortillas in sauce and place in the bottom of a 9 x 13 pan, sprayed with cooking spray. Take ⅓ of the chicken and spread over the first layer of tortillas. Sprinkle ½ cup of the shredded cheese over the chicken.
4. Dip 6 more tortillas in sauce and make a second layer in pan. Put the potato, pepper, and onion mixture onto the second layer of tortillas with ⅓ chicken, ½ cup cheese.
5. Dip 6 tortillas in sauce and layer in pan. Top with remaining chicken, ½ cup cheese.
6. Dip last 6 tortillas in sauce and place on top. Spoon any remaining sauce over the tortillas. Sprinkle with remaining cheese. Bake at 350 degrees for 20 minutes or until cheese is melted and hot.
7. Slice into squares to serve, topped with non-fat plain yogurt and chopped onions.

Servings: 12. **Nutrition Facts**: Serving size: ¹⁄₁₂ of a recipe (7 ounces), Amount Per Serving: Calories 313, Total Fat 10g, Saturated Fat 5g, Cholesterol 59mg, Sodium 371mg, Potassium 449mg, Total Carbohydrates 32g, Fiber 4g, Sugar 2g, Protein 22g

Food Group Servings = 1 Vegetable, 2 Grain, 2 Meat, 1.5 fats

Health Coach Tips:
- ♥ To save time, bake extra chicken for previous night's dinner to use for this meal.
- ♥ Use more seasonings to kick up the flavor. You can add more pepper, garlic powder, or chili powder to the chicken after you have chopped it up or a sweet chopped onion and fresh minced garlic. Top with Pico de Gallo or fresh salsa for even more flavor.

Good for You Tamale Pie

My friend Susan's version of Tamale Pie is full of flavor and vegetables yet lower in fat than the traditional version. You can make it vegetarian by using soy crumbles or more chopped vegetables in place of the ground turkey.

1 tablespoon canola oil
1 pound lean ground turkey
1 onion, diced
One 4-ounce can green chilies, chopped
1 green or red bell pepper, diced
One 28- ounce can crushed tomatoes
2 cups frozen corn
One 11-ounce can black olives
One 15-ounce can low-sodium kidney
    beans, rinsed and drained

2 ¼ cups yellow cornmeal
1 teaspoon salt
1 teaspoon cumin
2 teaspoons chili powder
¾ cup sharp cheddar cheese, shredded
1 ½ cup fat-free milk
2 cups water
2 tablespoons Smart Balance
1 teaspoon garlic powder (or 1 Tablespoon
    chopped fresh garlic)

1. Preheat oven to 400 degrees. Spray a 9 x 13 dish with cooking spray.
2. **To make your crust**: In a large saucepan, whisk 2 cups of cornmeal into 2 cups of cold water over medium heat. Add 1 teaspoon of salt and pepper to taste. Reduce heat and stir in milk, stirring often until mixture becomes thick, about 5 minutes. Stir in green chilies. Remove from heat and add in 2 Tablespoons trans fat free buttery spread.
3. Reserve 2 cups of the cornmeal to add to the filling. Spread remaining cornmeal on bottom of dish.
4. **To make your filling**: Heat 2 Tablespoons canola oil in a large nonstick skillet on medium heat. Brown ground turkey and onion, adding in spices, onion, and fresh peppers as it browns. Once meat is browned, add in tomatoes, chilies, corn, olives, and beans and remaining cornmeal mixture. Let simmer for about 5 minutes, stir well, and pour on top of cornmeal crust. Top with shredded cheese and bake about 20 minutes or until bubbly and golden brown.

Servings: 10

Nutrition Facts: Serving size: ¹⁄₁₀ of a recipe (11.7 ounces), Amount Per Serving: Calories 307, Total Fat 9g, Saturated Fat 3g, Cholesterol 26mg, Sodium 816mg, Potassium 566mg, Total Carbohydrates 42g, Fiber 6g, Sugar 7g, Protein 17g

Food Group Servings: 1 Serving = 1 Vegetable, 2 Grains, 1 Meat, 1 Beans, 1 fat

Health Coach Tip: Serve with a tossed green salad. To reduce sodium omit the olives or use low-sodium on all the canned items.

Heart Healthy Chili

You can whip up this chili in less than 20 minutes and tastes as good as homemade chili with beef. If you use ground beef, buy the leanest possible and rinse off the fat in a strainer with water after browning. Or you can use soy crumbles from the freezer, lean ground turkey or chicken. Choose options where you control the amount of fat.

1 medium bell pepper, chopped
1 Tablespoon Extra-virgin Olive Oil
One 11-ounce can pinto beans
One can black beans, drained
1 large can crushed tomatoes
One 11-ounce kidney, or white cannellini beans
1 cup soy TVP – Textured Vegetable Protein
(Bob's Red Mill Dried) or 1 cup lentils

1 tablespoon "No salt" seasoning
1 cup chicken broth, vegetable broth
or water
1 large yellow onion, peeled and
chopped
4 cloves garlic minced
2 tablespoons chili powder
2 tablespoons cumin

1. If you use ground beef, chicken or turkey sauté until brown, pour off any fat, then begin with the next step.
2. Chop the onion, bell pepper and sauté in a large heavy pot in olive oil on medium heat.
3. Add drained pinto, kidney, and black beans to onion and peppers. Stir in minced garlic.
4. Pour in crushed tomatoes and cup of chicken or vegetable broth. Stir well. Add in 1 cup of soy protein and seasonings, stirring well over medium heat. Add a little more broth if it is too thick. If you like your chili spicier, add more chili powder and cumin. Let simmer for a few minutes until the vegetables have cooked and flavors have absorbed. Top with such items as sliced green onions, grated cheddar cheese, low-fat sour cream, or fat-free plain yogurt. ***Remember every ounce of cheddar cheese adds about 9 grams of fat.***

Servings: 7

Nutrition Facts: Serving size: ⅐ of a recipe (10.9 ounces), Amount Per Serving: Calories 219, Total Fat 5, Saturated Fat .78g, Cholesterol 0mg, Sodium 566mg, Potassium 960mg, Total Carbohydrates 32g, Fiber 11g, Sugar 8g, Protein 15g

Food Group Servings: 1 Serving = 1 Vegetable, 2 Meat/Bean, 1 fat

Health Coach Tip:
♥ This chili is loaded with fiber and nutrients. For more veggies and flavor, add more fresh chopped tomatoes or more peppers such as poblanos, or jalapenos for more heat. Use your left over chili for dinner another night as a topping for baked potatoes or tamales.

Lighter Macaroni and Cheese

Mac n cheese can be good for you when you reduce the saturated fat, and add veggies and fiber. Try using multigrain pasta for even more nutrition.

4 slices 100% grain bread
¼ teaspoon salt
⅛ teaspoon pepper
1 ½ cups 1% milk
1 pound pasta shells
1 cup Parmigiano-Reggiano cheese

2 teaspoons unsalted butter
¾ cup cheddar cheese grated
2 teaspoons flour
¼ teaspoon black pepper
1 cup frozen green peas thawed
2 teaspoons Smart Balance or Earth Balance

1. Pulse bread in food processor until mixture resembles coarse crumbs to make about 1 ½ cups. Transfer to a small bowl, stir in ¼ cup of the parmesan cheese. Set aside.
2. Adjust oven rack to middle and preheat oven to 375 degrees.
3. Bring 4 quarts of water to a rolling boil in a stockpot. Combine cheese in large bowl; set aside. Add pasta and 1 Tablespoon salt to boiling water, stir in pasta.
4. While pasta is cooking, melt butter in small saucepan over medium-low heat; whisk flour into butter until no lumps remain, about 30 seconds. Gradually whisk in milk, increase heat to medium and bring to a boil, stirring occasionally; reduce heat to medium-low and simmer 1 minute to ensure flour cooks.
5. Stir in remaining ¼ teaspoon salt and pepper, cover milk mixture and set aside.
6. When pasta is done, al dente, drain and add to a large mixing bowl. Pour in cheese sauce and peas, and then gently mix to coat pasta.
7. Transfer pasta mixture to a 13 x 9 baking dish that has been sprayed with cooking spray. Sprinkle evenly with reserved bread crumbs then dot with 2 teaspoons of margarine.
8. Bake at 375 degrees about 20-30 minutes until hot. Serve immediately.

Servings: 8

Nutrition Facts: Serving size: ⅛ of a recipe (5.6 ounces), Amount Per Serving: Calories 392, Total Fat 11g, Saturated Fat 6, Cholesterol 28mg, Sodium 445mg, Potassium 239mg, Total Carbohydrates 54.12g, Fiber 2.61g, Sugar 4g, Protein 19g

Food Group Servings: 1 Serving = 1 grains, 1 dairy, 1 fat

Health Coach Tip:
♥ Pasta is a comfort food that does not have to be banished from the heart healthy or diabetic's meal plan. Whole wheat and whole grain pastas such as Barilla Pasta Plus are a delicious alternative, naturally rich in fiber, which slows the absorption of sugar and has minerals such as magnesium that increase the body's sensitivity to insulin. Remember to eat the correct portion size and fill in with vegetables.

Quick & Healthy Greek Pasta Dinner

Loaded with veggies, beans and protein, this quick dinner helps you to fit in servings from multiple food groups. Use multigrain pasta with more protein, Omega-3's and more fiber than regular pasta.

1 large onion chopped

Two 15- ounce cans tomatoes, diced

2 medium zucchini grated

8 ounces chicken broth with no msg

½ cup red or white wine

½ teaspoon salt and pepper to taste

1 pound Barilla Plus-Farfalle Multigrain Pasta

1 medium yellow bell pepper, chopped

1 medium red bell pepper, chopped

4 cloves garlic clove, minced

1 tablespoon Extra-virgin Olive Oil

1 pound lean ground turkey

1 can chickpeas, garbanzo beans, drained

½ teaspoon basil

1 teaspoon oregano

1. Cook pasta in boiling water according to directions while you start your sauce.
2. Heat olive oil in large deep skillet over medium heat. Add onions and sauté a couple of minutes, and then add ground turkey. Brown the turkey and add seasonings. Add wine to deglaze the pan, and then add the peppers and zucchini. Stir and let cook for a couple of minutes more before adding the tomatoes, red wine and chicken broth.
3. Add the garbanzo beans and stir the sauce. Let all the flavors come together and reduce down for a few minutes.
4. Add pasta and toss with your meat and vegetable sauce in the pot. Serve sprinkled with freshly grated parmesan cheese.

Servings: 8

Nutrition Facts: Serving size: ⅛ of a recipe (12 ounces), Amount Per Serving: Calories 167, Total Fat 5g, Saturated Fat 1g, Cholesterol 23mg, Sodium 553mg, Potassium 636mg, Total Carbohydrates 35, Fiber 6g, Sugar 7g, Protein 17g

Food Group Servings: 1 Serving = 2 vegetable, 1 grains, 1meat/bean

Health Coach Tip:
- ♥ You can add more seasonings to your taste. Serve with a green salad.

State Fair Tacos

When we were children, we would eat these delicious soft tacos at the California State Fair. They are simple, yet we've never forgotten the taste. I created the closest recipe possible. Steaming the tortillas saves on extra fat and calories. Serve with beans and sliced red onions.

1 pound lean ground beef
10 corn tortillas (about 6 -inches)
1 Tablespoon cumin
½ teaspoon salt and pepper to taste

1 head romaine lettuce, shredded
1 medium yellow onion, peeled, chopped
1 Tablespoon chili powder

1. Sauté lean ground beef in a large skillet until almost browned, then rinse in colander to remove all fat. Add beef back to skillet and finish browning with onions and spices.
2. In the meantime, steam tortillas to soften. Add in romaine lettuce to beef mixture and stir until mixed well. Put ground beef mixture in tortillas and roll up.

Servings: 10: **Nutrition Facts**: Serving size: ¹⁄₁₀ of a recipe (1 taco), Amount Per Serving: Calories 198, Total Fat 10g, Saturated Fat 4g, Cholesterol 34mg, Sodium 49mg, Potassium 356mg, Carbohydrates 16g, Fiber 3g, Sugar 1g, Protein 11g

Food Group Servings: 1 Serving = 1 Grains, 1 Meat, 2 Oils & Fats

Heart Healthy Spicy Soy Tacos

8 corn tortillas-6"
3 fresh tomatoes
8 ounces soy cheddar cheese
½ cup chopped onion (white or red)
¾ cup salsa
2 tablespoons minced, wet garlic

8 ounces vegetarian soy crumbles
cooking spray or butter substitute
4 green onions, washed & sliced
8 tablespoons nonfat, plain Greek yogurt
1 tablespoon chili powder

1. Spray tortillas with cooking spray or butter substitute spray. Line a cookie sheet with foil. Lay the tortillas on the foil and cover tightly with another sheet of foil. Warm the tortillas in the oven at 350 for 5 minutes just before serving.
2. Brown the soy crumbles in a skillet with ½ cup chopped onion, ¼ cup salsa and seasonings until onions are soft and everything is hot.
3. While the soy mixture is cooking, chop the green onions, tomatoes. Grate the soy cheese and build your taco bar with toppings: green onions, tomatoes, salsa, fat-free plain yogurt.

Spoon soy mixture into warm tortillas and fill with all your toppings. To stay at 5 grams of fat per taco, each taco only has 1 oz. of soy cheese and 1 tbsp of yogurt or sour cream.

Servings: 8 servings (1 taco)**Nutrition Facts:** Per Serving: 190 calories, fat 5 g, cholesterol 0 mg, sodium 630 mg, carbohydrates 22 g, fiber 5 g, sugar 4 g, protein 14 g

Food Group Portions: 1 protein, 1 grain

Stuffed Bell Peppers

The original stuffed bell peppers recipe used ground beef where the fat soaked into the rice. This cooking method has much less fat by substituting lean ground turkey or chicken for the beef and including more vegetables for flavor.

8 large red or green bell peppers
2 cups brown rice cooked
One 11-ounce can pinto beans or black beans
1 cup frozen corn
1 teaspoon chili powder
1 teaspoon cumin
1 teaspoon garlic salt, garlic powder or minced garlic

One 15-ounce can crushed tomatoes
1 cup mild or medium salsa
1 yellow onion, peeled and chopped
½ cup white wine
½ cup water
1 teaspoon Mrs. Dash no salt seasoning
1 pound chicken breasts ground or lean ground turkey, *browned with onions*

1. Preheat oven to 350 degrees.
2. Wash peppers, slice caps off, remove seeds. Slice usable parts of bell pepper caps.
3. Brown ground chicken or turkey with onions, pinch of salt and pepper.
4. In a large bowl combine chopped peppers, onions, beans, corn, rice, salsa, and ½ of the tomatoes. Mix with browned meat. Lightly pack mixture into bell peppers.
5. Place stuffed peppers into 13 x 9 x 2 inch baking dish. Pour remaining tomatoes over peppers. Sprinkle with 1 Tablespoon "no salt" seasoning. Pour ½ cup white wine over peppers and ½ cup water into the baking dish. Tent with foil.
6. Bake at 350 degrees for about 30 minutes until hot and bubbling. Make sure the bell peppers and poultry are thoroughly cooked.

Servings: 8

Nutrition Facts: Serving size: ⅛ of a recipe (20.1 ounces), Amount Per Serving: Calories 271,Total Fat 4g, Saturated Fat .47g, Cholesterol 33mg, Sodium 721mg, Potassium 859mg, Total Carbohydrates 40g, Fiber 9g, Sugar 2g, Protein 21g

Food Group Servings: 1 ½ vegetables, 1 grains, 2 meat/bean

Health Coach Tip:
- ♥ To give this a Mexican food flavor add cumin, chili powder and stuff poblano peppers instead of bell peppers. To keep it more traditional, use paprika and no salt seasoning. Use regular bell peppers, red, green and orange for color! Beautiful and delicious!

Baked Lentil Soup

This delicious soup recipe from my friend Joyce is a breeze to make! Throw everything in one covered pot; put it in the oven and less than two hours later dinner has made itself.

1 cup lentils

2 cups water

1 cup carrots, washed, peeled and sliced

1 cup celery diced

½ cup onion, chopped

1 large clove of garlic minced

1 can beef broth, or vegetable broth

One 8-ounce can tomato sauce

2 bay leaves

salt

1. Rinse lentils and drain. Combine water, lentils, celery, broth, tomato sauce, onion, garlic, bay leaves, salt and pepper in oven proof casserole.
2. Cover and bake at 350 degrees for 1 ½ to 2 hours.
3. Serve with toppings such as fat-free plain sour cream or yogurt, sliced green onions, and thinly sliced radishes.

Servings: 6

Nutrition Facts: 8 oz. per serving. Amount per serving: Calories 67, Total fat 0.38, Cholesterol 0, Sodium 377mg, Carbohydrates 12, Fiber 4, Sugar 4g, Protein 4g.

Food Group Servings: 1 Serving = ½ vegetable, 1 legume/protein.

Health Coach Tip*:*
♥ When preparing the soup, you can also add other vegetables you have on hand such as sliced mushrooms, bell peppers or zucchini to increase the number of vegetables to count toward your daily total. The more vegetables the better!

Best Meatloaf or Meatless ~ You Choose

This original recipe came from my friend Phyllis. It works with lean ground beef, lean ground turkey, or soy crumbles in the frozen health food section of your grocery store or use dry TVP- *Textured Vegetable Protein*- rehydrated.

1 onion finely chopped	1 teaspoon garlic powder
2 stalks celery finely chopped	1 teaspoon season salt, ½ teas. pepper
2 carrots, peeled and finely chopped	¼ cup ketchup
2 tomatoes, diced	2 tablespoons vinegar
2 tablespoons Worcestershire sauce	1 teaspoon Dijon mustard
1 cup oats	2 eggs beaten
½ cup 1% milk	1 pound lean ground beef or TVP or crumbles
1 cup oatmeal	2 Tablespoons brown sugar (packed)

1. Spray a 9 x 13 pan with cooking spray. Preheat oven to 350 degrees.
2. In a large bowl combine vegetarian soy crumbles or TVP or ground beef or ground turkey, onion, celery, carrots, tomatoes, eggs, Worcestershire sauce, season salt, garlic powder, pepper, oats and milk. Toss lightly and set aside.
3. Make a topping by mixing the ketchup, mustard, brown sugar and vinegar.
4. Form the "meatloaf" into a rectangle about two inches thick and place in 9 x 13 pan.
5. Spread topping over loaf. Bake at 350 for about one hour or until no longer pink on inside. *Let stand a few minutes before serving with mashed potatoes or mashed cauliflower and a green vegetable.*

Servings: 8

Nutrition Facts for Lean Ground Beef Meatloaf : Serving size: ⅛ of a recipe (7 ounces), Per serving: Calories 274, **Total Fat 14g**, Saturated Fat 5g, Cholesterol 96g, Sodium 492mg, Potassium 487mg, Total Carbohydrates 22g, Fiber 2g, Sugar 10g, Protein 15g
Nutrition Facts for Lean Ground Turkey Meatloaf : Serving size: ⅛ of a recipe (7 ounces), Per serving: Calories 193, **Total Fat 3g**, Saturated Fat 1g, Cholesterol 24, Sodium 810mg, Potassium 504mg, Total Carbohydrates 22g, Fiber 2g, Sugar 10g, Protein 15g
Nutrition Facts for Vegetarian loaf : Serving size: ⅛ of a recipe (7 ounces), Amount Per Serving: Calories 161, **Total Fat 1g**, Saturated Fat 0.39g, Cholesterol 1.2mg, Sodium 450 mg, Potassium 687mg, Total Carbohydrates 26g, Fiber 5g, Sugar 12g, Protein 12g

Food Group Serving: 1 Vegetable, 1 meat/beans.

Notice the difference in the nutrition facts on each type of loaf!

Very Veggie Sides

~

Apple Cinnamon Roasted Butternut Squash

1 lb. butternut squash peeled, cut 1 into inch cubes
1 medium apple, diced
2 tablespoons Smart Balance or Earth Balance
2 tablespoons honey

¼ cup pecans, chopped
½ teaspoon nutmeg
½ teaspoon cinnamon

1. Preheat oven to 400 degrees.
2. Places cubed squash and apple in an 8x8 baking dish sprayed with cooking spray. Add 3 Tablespoons of water and roast uncovered, stirring occasionally for 20 minutes, or almost cooked through.
3. Meanwhile, in a small bowl, combine next five ingredients.
4. Remove squash from oven and pour honey mix over squash. Stir lightly to coat. Return to the oven for 10 minutes more or until cooked through.
5. Remove from oven and serve in a serving dish or around roast pork or chicken.

Servings: 6

Nutrition Facts: Serving size: ⅙ of a recipe (4.1 ounces), Amount Per Serving: Calories 115.87, Total Fat 5, Saturated Fat 1g, Cholesterol 0mg, Sodium 31mg, Potassium 316mg, Total Carbohydrates 19g, Fiber 3g, Sugar 10g, Protein 1g

Food Group Servings= 1 Vegetable, 1 fat

Health Coach Tips:
♥ Butternut squash is sweet, buttery tasting and full of fiber that provides a full feeling and also slows down the rise in blood sugar levels. Beta-carotene, the antioxidant form of vitamin A helps maintain eye health and promotes healthy skin.
♥ Pecans can help protect you from heart disease. Studies have shown that just a few ounces of pecans daily can reduce triglyceride and LDL cholesterol levels. Pecans contain vitamin E which helps prevent damage to heart blood vessels. They also have potassium, calcium and magnesium to help lower blood pressure.

Lighter Potato Salad

I changed my mother's famous potato salad recipe by lightening it up and reducing the fat and everyone still loves it.

10 medium potatoes, red or Yukon gold, unpeeled, wash and diced medium size
½ cup celery, chopped fine in food processor
1 cup red onion, chopped fine
¼ cup parsley chopped
2 eggs
Salt and pepper, to taste

8 tomato slices
¼ cup mayonnaise
¼ cup plain, fat-free plain yogurt
1 tablespoon lemon juice
4 tablespoons red wine vinegar
1 tablespoon Dijon-style mustard

1. Boil the potatoes unpeeled until fork tender, but not mushy about 10-15 minutes. Add the eggs to hard boil while the potatoes are cooking the last 10 minutes. Drain the potatoes. Cool the eggs in cold water. Put them in a large bowl.
2. Sprinkle warm potatoes with 3 Tablespoons vinegar and ½ teaspoon salt and ¼ teaspoon of pepper. Chop the celery, onion, and parsley in a food processor. Add to the potatoes. Peel and grate the hard-boiled eggs with a cheese grater. Add to the potatoes.
3. In a small bowl, mix the mayonnaise, yogurt, lemon juice, mustard, and one Tablespoon of the vinegar.
4. Toss the potatoes with the onions, celery and eggs gently. Fold in the dressing and toss gently. Taste the salad at this point. If you need to add more salt, pepper, vinegar or other seasoning. Then toss again. Transfer to a serving bowl, surround with tomato slices. Garnish top with parsley and paprika.

Servings: 16

Nutrition Facts: Serving size: 9 ounces (approx. 1 cup) Amount Per Serving: Calories 144, Total Fat 2g, Saturated Fat 0.4g, Cholesterol 28mg, Sodium 68mg, Potassium 717mg, Total Carbohydrates 25g, Fiber 4g, Sugar 4g, Protein 4g

Food Group Servings= 1 Vegetable, 1 fat

Health Coach Tip:
♥ To cut down on fat and cholesterol leave out the egg yolks and use low-fat mayonnaise. Best Foods light mayonnaise has only 1 gram of fat, is low in calories and tastes good. You can also use buttermilk in place of the mayonnaise or yogurt for a more creamy texture.

Tea Garlic Sesame Greens

Add antioxidant packed green tea to your stir-fry. Sesame seeds and garlic add flavor too.

1 Tablespoon extra virgin olive oil

1 teaspoon chili powder or 21 seasoning

1 pound fresh spinach and kale, washed and stems removed

¼ teaspoon salt

2 cups cooked brown rice

2 teaspoons green tea

3 cloves garlic, minced

2 Tablespoons sesame seeds

¼ teaspoon pepper

1. Prepare 2 cups of brown rice as directed on package.
2. While rice is cooking, heat oil in a Dutch oven over medium high heat. Add tea, chili powder or veggie seasoning, and garlic, stirring for 30 seconds.
3. Add spinach and stir-fry for 2 minutes.
4. Stir in vinegar and cook for 1 minute more until spinach wilts.
5. Sprinkle with sesame seeds, salt, and pepper. Serve over brown rice.

Servings: 4

Nutrition Facts: Serving size: ¼ of a recipe (9.6 ounces), Amount Per Serving: Calories 199, Total Fat 8g, Saturated Fat .83g, Cholesterol 0mg, Sodium 243mg, Potassium 7542mg, Total Carbohydrates 29g, Fiber 5g, Sugar .56g, Protein 6g

Food Group Servings= 1 Vegetable, 1 fats, 1 grains

Health Coach Tips:
- ♥ Greens are great! Add other greens such as cabbage, Bok Choy, asparagus and Swiss chard as all are highly nutritious. Kale and leafy greens are low in calories and high in fiber which is great for digestion. They are also filled with folate, magnesium, iron and Vitamin K which can help protect against various cancers. Kale is a great anti-inflammatory food filled with 10% of the RDA of omega-3 fatty acids, which help, fight against arthritis, asthma and autoimmune disorders. Greens can help lower cholesterol when prepared without fats like bacon. Lastly greens are high in calcium which helps prevent osteoporosis.
- ♥ You can find salt free seasonings everywhere. Mrs. Dash, Bragg's and Costco make a flavorful seasoning blend that adds vibrant flavor to all vegetables.
- ♥ *Brown rice takes about 45 minutes or more to cook depending on the variety. Plan ahead and cook it the night before or on the weekend when you have more time, making this a quick dinner.*

Pecan Sweet Potatoes

This is a great side dish. To save on calories and sugar, you can omit the topping and simply put chopped or whole pecans on top. Save leftovers to make a sweet potato snack cake.

6 sweet potatoes and 6 yams
2 eggs
2 Tablespoons Smart Balance
½ cup 1% milk
¼ cup orange juice
½ teaspoon salt

1 Tablespoon vanilla
Topping:
¼ cup brown sugar
¼ cup whole wheat flour
2 Tablespoons buttery spread
¾ cup chopped pecans

1. Wash sweet potatoes and or yams, pat dry and roast for about 45 minutes or until tender. Let cool slightly and peel most of the skin off.
2. In a large mixing bowl, combine yams and sweet potatoes, eggs, milk, orange juice, margarine, salt and vanilla. Place in a casserole dish that has been sprayed with cooking spray.
3. Melt buttery spread. Combine topping ingredients in a small bowl. Pour butter over topping ingredients and stir. Spread topping over yams. Bake at 350 degrees for about 30 minutes or until hot.

Servings: 8.

Nutrition Facts: Serving size: ⅛ of a recipe (6 ounces), Amount Per Serving: Calories 245, Total Fat 14g, Saturated Fat 7g, Cholesterol 61mg, Sodium 181mg, Potassium 361mg, Total Carbohydrates 26g, Fiber 3g, Sugar 11g, Protein 4g

Food Group Servings= 1 Vegetable, ½ nut/seed, 1 fat

Health Coach Tips:
- Sweet potatoes and yams are different, yet both stabilize blood sugar levels which aid in management of diabetes and weight. Both have fiber which helps us to feel full longer. They also supply vitamin A and C to help fight infection and lower blood pressure.
- The easiest way to prepare them is to wash and roast them whole. Leave the peel on to gain additional nutrients. Add roasted sweet potatoes and yams to your muffins and quick breads to add moisture and nutrition.

Quinoa, Brown Rice & Mandarin Orange Salad

Quinoa is classified by the National Academy of Sciences as one of the best sources of protein and the only grain that provides all the eight essential amino acids. *(It is technically a seed that behaves like a grain.)* Each serving provides 3 grams of fiber and 6 grams of proteins, making it ideal for vegetarians.

1 cup quinoa

1 cup brown rice

1 cup snow peas

1 cup each red & yellow bell pepper diced

½ cup golden raisins

½ cup red onion diced

½ cup almonds chopped or slivered

1 cup Mandarin oranges

2 tablespoons vinegar

2 tablespoons olive oil

2 tablespoons orange juice

1. Cook quinoa according to directions on package with water.
2. Cook brown rice according to directions on package.
3. Wash and slice sugar snap peas or snow peas into thirds. Dice onions and sweet peppers. Wash and thinly slice green onions.
4. When rice and quinoa are cooked and cooled, put them in a large bowl. Add all the chopped vegetables, mandarins, almonds, and onions.
5. Whisk vinegar and oil with a little salt and pepper to taste. Add 1 teaspoon of sugar if desired. Toss the rice salad with the dressing and raisins. Chill or serve at room temperature.

Servings: 8

Nutrition Facts: Serving size: ⅛ of a recipe (5.6 ounces), Amount Per Serving: Calories 242, Total Fat 9g, Saturated Fat 1g, Cholesterol 0mg, Sodium 150mg, Potassium 414mg, Total Carbohydrates 35g, Fiber 5g, Sugar 9g, Protein 7g

Food Group Servings = ½ Vegetable, 1 ½ grains, 2 fats

Health Coach Tips:
- Prepare your brown rice ahead of time, as it takes longer to cook than the quinoa. If you can find brown basmati rice, it has a nice light quality.
- Snow's Citrus makes a great mandarin orange dressing if you don't want to make your own. www.snowscitrus.com.

Summer Squash and Veggie Sauté

This dish is very easy to prepare on a hot summer day.

1 white, yellow, purple or green onions
2 zucchini, sliced in thin rounds
2 summer squash, thinly sliced
2 yellow crook neck squash, thinly sliced
½ teaspoon salt and pepper to taste

2 cups fresh mushrooms, sliced
2 cups diced tomatoes
1 tablespoon extra-virgin olive oil
2 tablespoons Mrs. Dash no salt seasoning

1. Sauté one or more of any combination of vegetables in a small amount of olive oil in large skillet until tender. Add salt, pepper, and seasoning to taste.
2. For a splash of flavor, sprinkle with freshly grated parmesan cheese just before serving.

Servings: 6

Nutrition Facts: Serving size: ⅙ of a recipe (4.9 ounces), Amount Per Serving: Calories 61, Total Fat 4.09g, Saturated Fat <1, Cholesterol 0mg, Sodium 12mg, Potassium 347mg, Total Carbohydrates 5g, Fiber 2g, Sugar 2g, Protein 2g

Food Group Servings = 2 Vegetable

Health Coach Tip
♥ Seasonings such as Mrs. Dash, oregano and fresh garlic give this dish extra flavor. This is a high nutrient, low calorie dish that is so low in fat, calories and carbohydrates that you can eat quite a lot. When you eat lots of fresh vegetables you fill up on foods that benefit you while helping you maintain a healthy weight.

Sweet Orange Carrots

If you prefer apricot or peach, either jam will give the carrots a sweeter flavor, encouraging us to eat our beta-carotene which is proven to improve eyesight.

4 cups carrots, peeled and sliced
1 tablespoon butter or Smart Balance
2 tablespoons lemon juice

2 tablespoons orange marmalade or no sugar jam such as peach or apricot
Salt to taste, a pinch will do

1. In a 3 quart saucepan over high heat, bring 1 inch water to boil. Place carrots in steamer insert and set over water. Reduce heat to medium and steam, covered 8 minutes until tender. *If you don't have a steamer, cook in a small amount of water that will absorb while cooking.* Drain and toss with 1 Tablespoon butter or buttery spread.
2. Toss with marmalade and a pinch of salt if desired and serve. *Chopped pecans make a nice addition!*

Servings: 8

Nutrition Facts: Serving size: ⅛ of a recipe (2.6 ounces), Amount Per Serving: Calories 45, Total Fat >1g, Saturated Fat >1 Cholesterol 0mg, Sodium 57mg, Potassium 212mg, Total Carbohydrates 10g, Fiber 2g, Sugar 6, Protein>1g.

Food Group Serving = 1 Vegetable

Health Coach Tip:
- For best tasting carrots, make sure they are fresh true baby carrots, or buy fresh bulk carrots and slice, then cut them into rounds.
- Benefits of eating carrots: They are low in carbohydrates, high in Vitamin A, contain soluble fiber that helps you feel full and have one of the highest amounts of beta-carotene of any food to help defend from damage to the heart, blood vessels and eyes.
- Remember to add carrots to soups, sauces casseroles and quick breads.

Sweet Potato Not Fries

Try this easy, delicious, nutritious and healthy alternative to French fried potatoes or fried sweet potatoes. Roasting the sweet potatoes ahead of time allows you to make this quickly during your week.

6 sweet potatoes, yams mixed   Salt and pepper to taste
2 Tablespoons canola oil

1. Wash and pat dry sweet potatoes and or yams. Peel off any bad spots, but leave the rest of the peels as that is where much of the nutrition is.
2. Place sweet potatoes in a 9 x 13 or other baking dish and sprinkle with salt and pepper. Drizzle with 1 Tablespoon of the canola oil and rub all over.
3. Bake at 350 degrees for one to one and a half hours until fork tender. Cool.
4. Slice potatoes into ½ inch rounds and place into a heavy skillet with 1 Tablespoon of the canola oil. Lightly salt and pepper if desired.
5. Sauté in the skillet until browned. Serve as a side dish instead of deep fried French fries or chips. (*They don't come out as crispy as fries, but they aren't full of fat either.*)

Servings: 6

Nutrition Facts: Serving size: ⅙ of a recipe (4.8 ounces), Amount Per Serving: Calories 153 Total Fat 5g, Saturated Fat >1g, Cholesterol 0mg, Sodium 72mg, Potassium 438mg, Total Carbohydrates 26g, Fiber 4g, Sugar 5g, Protein 2g

Food Group Servings = 1 Vegetable, 1 fats

Health Coach Tip:
♥ Roast the sweet potatoes when you have time, then cool and keep them in the refrigerator. You can pull them out and cook this delicious side dish in minutes.

Yogurt and Cucumber Salad

2 cucumbers, sliced into ¼ inch slices
½ red onion
3 cloves garlic, minced
Salt and pepper to taste

3 cloves garlic, minced
1 tablespoon extra virgin olive oil
2 cups low fat plain yogurt

1. Slice the cucumbers into rounds. Place in a colander to get rid of excess water.
2. Peel and slice the red onion as thinly as possible.
3. Place the yogurt in a large salad bowl; add the garlic, salt, and pepper to taste. Mix well.
4. Add the cucumbers and onion slices, and then drizzle on the oil. Serve chilled.

Servings: 6

Nutrition Facts: Serving size: ⅙ of a recipe (6.8 ounces), Amount Per Serving: Calories 86, Total Fat 4g, Saturated Fat 1g, Cholesterol 4mg, Sodium 56mg, Potassium 323.63mg, Total Carbohydrates 8g, Fiber >1g, Sugar 1g, Protein 5g

Food Group Servings = 1 Vegetable, 1 milk,

Health Coach Tips:
- ♥ Yogurt is a beneficial food for anyone who wants to prevent heart disease, diabetes or who has diabetes. Yogurt is a nutrient rich substitute for higher calorie, sugary desserts and helps battle hunger by stabilizing blood sugar.
- ♥ Yogurt, especially non-fat Greek yogurt is high in protein (although slightly lower in calcium) and can be substituted for high fat meats. The live active bacteria cultures in yogurt help with digestive health by suppressing the growth of harmful bacteria in the intestinal tract. These beneficial bacteria promote strong immune function.

Zucchini Patties

Those of us who grow vegetable gardens have an overabundance of zucchini each summer. This recipe is a tasty way to eat up all that nutritious squash.

4 cups grated zucchini
1 bunch green onions, sliced
2 tablespoons fresh Italian parsley
2 eggs slightly beaten

1 tablespoon paprika
½ cup crumbled feta cheese
1 cup all-purpose flour or whole wheat
4 tablespoons extra virgin olive oil

1. Grate zucchini in food processor for fastest preparation. Place zucchini in a colander, sprinkle with salt and let drain for 15 minutes to remove excess moisture.
2. Put the drained zucchini is a large bowl with the green onions, parsley, eggs, and paprika, mixing well. Add a sprinkle of salt and pepper. Stir in the feta cheese and flour a little at a time until incorporated.
3. Heat oil in a skillet, and then lower to medium. Scoop out in ¼ spoonfuls into hot pan. Cook until golden brown on one side, then flip over and cook about 5 minutes on each side, making sure they are done all the way through. Drain on paper towels.
4. Serve at once with Garlic Yogurt Sauce or serve them at room temperature.

Servings: 12. **Nutrition Facts**: Serving size: ¹⁄₁₂ of a recipe (2.8 ounces), Amount Per Serving: Calories 118, Total Fat 7g, Saturated Fat 2g, Cholesterol 41mg, Sodium 89mg, Potassium 181mg, Total Carbohydrates 10.72g, Fiber 1.25g, Sugar 1.34g, Protein 3.81g

Food Group Servings = 1 Vegetable, 1 fat

Health Coach Tip:
♥ Before cooking each batch, stir the batter to prevent the patties from getting watery. *Garlic Yogurt Sauce is a great topping for the patties.*

Garlic Yogurt Sauce

1 ⅔ cup low fat plain yogurt   4 cloves garlic, minced

Salt to taste

1. In a small bowl, whisk the yogurt, garlic, and salt until the mixture is very smooth.
2. Cover and refrigerate for at least 15 minutes before serving.

Servings: 10.

Nutrition Facts: Serving size: ¹⁄₁₀ of a recipe (1.5 ounces), Amount Per Serving: Calories 27.51, Total Fat 1g, Saturated Fat >1g, Cholesterol 2mg, Sodium 36mg, Potassium 100mg, Total Carbohydrates 3g, Fiber .03g, Sugar 3g, Protein 2.g

Food Group Serving=1Milk

Health Coach Tip: This sauce is good on plain cooked leafy green spinach or chard.

Mashed Cauliflower

Mashed cauliflower tastes similar to mashed potatoes but with fewer carbohydrates, low in sugars and starches so it won't cause your blood sugar to spike. You can also make half cauliflower and half mashed potatoes for a satisfying side dish.

1 head cauliflower, cut into small pieces	Salt and pepper to taste
1 tablespoon extra virgin olive oil	Freshly grated parmesan cheese, optional

1. Bring a large pot of salted water to a boil. Add cauliflower and cook until tender, about 10 minutes. Reserve ¼ cup of the cooking liquid and then drain well and transfer cauliflower to a food processor or mixer. Add olive oil and reserved water, 1 tablespoon at a time and puree until smooth. You can also mash with a potato masher. Sprinkle with salt and pepper and freshly grated parmesan cheese if you like.

Servings: 4

Nutrition Facts: Serving size: ¼ of recipe. Amount per servings: Calories 110, Total fat 9g, saturated fat 1 g, cholesterol 0mg, Sodium 330, Carbohydrate 8g, Dietary Fiber 3 g, Sugar 3 g, Protein 3g.

Food Group Servings: 1 vegetable, 1 fat

Health Coach Tips:
- Cauliflower can be described as a *superfood*. It is a member of the cruciferous family of vegetables that have been shown to prevent cancer. Research has been show that combining cauliflower with curcumin, the active compound in the spice turmeric, may help prevent and treat prostate cancer.
- **Cauliflower benefits** heart health by improving blood pressure and kidney function. It is anti-inflammatory which helps your body prevent diseases. It is rich in vitamins, minerals such as Vitamin C, Vitamin K, B6, and many more. Cauliflower is a good source of choline, a B vitamin that helps with brain development and boosting cognitive brain function. It is also a good source of fiber for digestive health. It is full of antioxidants and phytonutrients which are nature's way of protecting you your cells against chronic stress and free radicals.

Refreshing Pineapple Carrot Raisin Salad

This is not your grandmother's carrot salad. It is light and fresh because it doesn't contain mayonnaise. Everyone loves it.

1 ½ pounds carrots, peeled and grated

1 tsp lemon juice

1 cup golden raisins

½ cup chopped walnuts or pecans

1 large can crushed pineapple

1 can mandarin oranges

¼ cup orange juice

1. Drain one half the juice from the pineapple and put in a large bowl with the other ingredients. Use a food processor to grate your carrots, making this salad a breeze. Toss well.

Servings: 8

Nutrition Facts: Serving size: ⅛ of recipe (6.1) ounces. Amount per servings: Calories 166, Total fat 5g, Saturated fat >1 g, Cholesterol 0mg, Sodium 62mg, Carbohydrate 31g, Dietary Fiber 4g, Sugar 21g, Protein 3g.

Food Group Servings: 1 vegetable, 1 fruit, 1 fat

Health Coach Tip:
♥ Eat pineapple to beat inflammation. Pineapple is rich in vitamin C and the enzyme bromelain, which has been linked to decreased pain and swelling in both osteoarthritis and rheumatoid arthritis. Pineapple also offers heart-protective folate and potassium which are needed for healthy blood pressure.
♥ Don't be afraid to buy and trim a fresh pineapple yourself. A ripe pineapple gives off a sweet aroma and is juicy, sweet and flavorful.

Curry Vegetables

2 cups broccoli florets
2 cups cauliflower florets
4 carrots sliced into ¼ inch rounds
2 medium zucchini, cut ½" slices
1 medium yellow onion, chopped
½ teaspoon salt and pepper to taste

1 tablespoon Extra Virgin Olive Oil
½ soy milk
1 cup water
1 teaspoon chicken style seasoning
1 tablespoon minced garlic
1 tablespoon Curry Powder

1. Place washed and cut vegetables into a large steamer and steam until tender.
2. In a large deep skillet sauté onions in olive oil until tender.
3. Whisk flour in a bowl in 1 cup water until blended and add to the skillet with the onions. Whisk in chicken bouillon or chicken style seasoning, garlic, salt and pepper. Heat to a boil to thicken sauce. Whisk in soy milk and stir until sauce is thickened. Stir in Curry Powder.
4. Add vegetables and fold into sauce carefully.
5. Serve on a large platter over couscous or brown rice.

Servings: 6

Nutrition Facts: Serving size: ⅙ of a recipe (9 ounces), Amount Per Serving: Calories 99, Total Fat 3 g, Saturated Fat >1g, Cholesterol 0mg, Sodium 135mg, Potassium 584mg, Total Carbohydrates Fiber 4g, Sugar 6g, Protein 4g

Food Group Servings = 2 Vegetable

Health Coach Tip:
♥ Curry, a mixed spice powder that is a staple of Indian cooking, may also have an array of health benefits. It contains turmeric, the spice that gives curry its familiar color and flavor. Studies concluded turmeric protects against several diseases. This food spice shows anti-inflammatory and antioxidant properties. Curcumin, a compound found in turmeric might improve symptoms of inflammation in many areas. Research shows that adding curry powder to your dishes may help keep you healthy.

Marcos' Potatoes

This recipe comes from Chef Marcos Maykall, who teamed with me to prepare meals for the Diabetes Prevention Program at our local health clinic. This method saves on calories and replaces fat and extra cheese, with potato and herb flavors. A real favorite and easy to make.

8 potatoes, Yukon gold or red	1 teaspoon rosemary
1 cup chicken broth, with no msg	1 teaspoon thyme
¼ cup Parmesan cheese, freshly grated	1 tablespoon smart balance margarine

1. Prepare a 9x12 glass baking dish with cooking spray. Preheat oven to 400 degrees.
2. Scrub and pat dry the potatoes. Slice the bottoms off so they will sit flat. Then slice each potato in ¼ inch slices, but hold them together as you place each potato in the baking dish. Push on the potatoes so they fall slightly like dominos to allow liquid to soak in.
3. Melt the smart balance in the microwave then mix in a bowl with the chicken broth and herbs. Pour over the potatoes.
4. Bake in the oven for 45 minutes or until tender. Remove from oven, sprinkle with parmesan cheese and bake for 5 minutes more or until the cheese is melted. Remove from the oven and sprinkle with black pepper and sliced green onions.

8 servings: ⅛ of the recipe (4.5 oz)

Per Serving: 117 calories, fat 2g, cholesterol 3mg, sodium 160mg, carbohydrates 22g, fiber 2g, sugar 0.12 g, protein 5g

Food Group Portions: 1 vegetable

Health Coach Tips:
- ♥ You save on calories and fat by preparing the potatoes this way instead of au gratin or cheesy methods. Everyone loves this fresh, flavorful, yet light way to prepare potatoes.
- ♥ Waxy potatoes like Yukon gold or red work best in this recipe as they hold together and have lots of flavor.
- ♥ Leaving the peel on provides fiber and helps slow digestion, keeping you full longer and limits the rise of blood sugar, making this a good dish for diabetics and pre-diabetics.
- ♥ Potatoes are packed with heart protective, immune-boosting vitamin C and blood pressure lowering potassium.

Satisfying Snacks & Appetizers

Snacks are an important part of your day because they prevent you from getting hungry and overeating at the next meal. A small healthy snack provides you with energy to get through the morning or mid-afternoon slump. *Here are a few tips for healthy snacks:*

1. If you aren't a big breakfast eater, split your healthy breakfast in half and save the rest for later in the morning. Yogurt, fruit and granola make great snacks.
2. When you have a snack, be mindful. Take a break and eat it slowly.
3. Eat a combination of a protein, fat and whole grain carbohydrate or fruit at the same time to help balance your blood sugar and help you feel full longer.

Almond Butter and Banana Sandwich

To cut calories, eat one half sandwich with an apple. Also makes a great after school or pre-game snack providing energy and protein to keep your kids going.

4 slices 100% whole grain bread
2 Tablespoons almond butter

1 banana, peeled and sliced
2 tablespoons honey

1. Spread almond butter evenly on two slices of bread. Spread honey on the other two slices.
2. Top slices of bread with sliced bananas and honey.
3. Enjoy with a glass of fat-free milk.

Servings: Makes 2 sandwiches. Serving sizes is one sandwich.

Nutrition Facts: Serving size: ½ of a recipe (5.1 ounces), Amount Per Serving: Calories 370, Total Fat 11g, Saturated Fat 1.42g, Cholesterol 0mg, Sodium 365mg, Potassium 506. mg, Total Carbohydrates 60g, Fiber 7g, Sugar 28g, Protein 11g

Food Group Servings: 1 Serving = 2 Grains, 1 nut, ½ fruit, 2 fats

Health Coach Tip:
♥ Bananas are rich with potassium and help to balance fluids in the body, helping to prevent leg cramps. Almond butter is an excellent source of healthy protein and good fat to keep you satisfied.

Blueberry & Dairy Snack

¼ cup fat-free cottage cheese
¼ cup fat-free yogurt, vanilla

½ cup blueberries
1 tablespoons walnuts, finely chopped

1. Take your nicest small bowl, put in cottage cheese, top with fat-free vanilla yogurt, blueberries, and chopped nuts.
2. Enjoy slowly...

Servings: 1

Nutrition Facts: Serving size: 1 of a recipe (4 ounces), Amount Per Serving: Calories 102, Total Fat 5g, Saturated Fat <1g, Cholesterol 3mg, Sodium 7mg, Potassium 109mg, Total Carbohydrates 12g, Fiber 2g, Sugar 8g, Protein 8g

Food Group Servings: 1 Serving = 1 Fruit, ½ milk, 1 nut/oil

Health Coach Tip: When you eat a snack that has protein, carbohydrates, and healthy fat, you will be satisfied until your next meal while getting valuable nutrition, instead of snacking on empty calories that leave you hungry and low on energy. When you snack, energize yourself on foods that fuel and nourish you.

Easy Berry Smoothie

You can make your smoothie with milk, soy milk, almond milk or Kefir which is a fermented drink full of vitamins and beneficial microorganisms that we need for a healthy gut. It tastes great alone or blended into a smoothie. Keeping frozen berries on hand makes blending a breeze.

2 cups fat-free kefir or 1 cup fat-free milk
6 ounces of fat-free strawberry or plain yogurt

1 cup strawberries, washed and halved
   or use frozen mixed berries

1. Place ingredients in a blender and mix well.

Serving size: 1

Nutrition Facts: Amount per serving: **C**alories 122, fat 0g, cholesterol 10 mg, sodium 258mg, carbohydrates 18g, fiber 2g, sugar 15 g, protein 9 g.

Food Group Servings: 2 servings of dairy, 1 fruit.

Health Coach Tips:
- Smoothies are a quick and delicious way to get nutrition, vitamins, minerals, protein, and energy in a hurry! Power pack your smoothie by adding powdered "greens" that you will find at the health food store, or add a cup of fresh spinach or kale. You do not taste the greens when using mixed berries, blueberries or apples.
- The variations are endless: blueberries, raspberries, bananas, oranges, use fruit that is in season. Add yogurt, protein powder, fat-free milk, almond milk or soy milk. Just measure your ingredients as you put them in the blender by calories or portion sizes so you know exactly how many calories or servings you are getting. Make your own tasty creations.

Brown Rice Veggie & Quinoa Cakes

This nutritious recipe can be served as an appetizer, snack, or side dish. What a delicious way to get fiber, protein, and B vitamins.

1 cup brown rice

½ cup quinoa, rinsed

2 ½ cups water

½ red bell pepper seeded and diced

4 teaspoons olive oil

6 medium green onions (scallions) sliced

2 medium carrots grated

½ cup pecans, chopped

4 ounces goat cheese

1 large egg white

1 teaspoon Mrs. Dash no salt seasoning

½ teaspoon salt and black pepper to taste

¼ red onion, minced

1. Rinse quinoa and brown rice and put in a large pan that has a tight fitting lid with water. Bring water to a boil, reduce heat to low, cover, and simmer at the lowest bubble until the water is absorbed and the rice and quinoa are tender, approximately 40 to 50 minutes. Remove from the heat and let stand covered for at least 10 minutes.
2. Preheat the oven to 400 degrees. Meanwhile, heat 2 teaspoons of the oil in a large skillet over medium heat. Add green onions, peppers, purple onion, and grated carrots. Sauté for a few minutes until tender. Remove from the heat.
3. Transfer the cooked vegetables, rice, and quinoa to a large food processor. Add pecans goat cheese, egg white, and seasonings. Pulse lightly until well blended but a little crumbly. Transfer mixture to a large bowl. Form the mixture into 2 inch patties. Makes about 14 cakes.
4. Heat the remaining 2 teaspoons oil in a large nonstick skillet over medium heat. Add the patties and cook about 3 to 4 minutes per side. Place rice cakes on a baking sheet sprayed with cooking spray and bake until golden brown about 10 to 15 minutes.

Servings: 14.

Nutrition Facts: Serving size: ¹⁄₁₄ of a recipe (4.9 ounces), Amount Per Serving: Calories 120, Total Fat 6g, Saturated Fat 2g, Cholesterol 4mg, Sodium 134mg, Potassium 235mg, Total Carbohydrates 14g, Fiber 2g, Sugar 2g, Protein 4.g

Food Group Servings: 1 Serving = 1 Vegetable, 1 grain, 1 fat

Health Coach Tip: Make a batch of brown rice and quinoa on the weekend, then you will have plenty on hand for the week to make quick rice cakes.

Cucumber Dip with Grilled Vegetables

For an even richer flavor, grill or roast vegetables such as asparagus and eggplant and let cool before serving.

½ cup plain nonfat yogurt
½ cup light sour cream
1 medium cucumber, peeled, and chopped

1 clove garlic, minced
1 Tablespoon minced fresh dill
Salt and pepper to taste

1. In medium bowl, combine sour cream and nonfat yogurt. Stir in cucumber, garlic, and dill. Season with salt and pepper. Arrange on a platter or vegetables by color.
2. Serve with assorted fresh or grilled vegetables such as carrot sticks, cucumber and mushroom slices, zucchini spears, red, green and or yellow bell pepper strips, celery stick, green onions and radish flowers. To grill, marinate your veggies in plastic bags with an oil and vinegar dressing, homemade or bottled, then place on the grill until slightly tender.

Servings: 6

Nutrition Facts: Serving size: ⅙ of recipe (3 ounces), Amount Per Serving: Calories 32 Total Fat 1g, Saturated Fat <1g, Cholesterol 5mg, Sodium 22mg, Potassium 134mg, Total Carbohydrates 3g, Fiber 1g, Sugar 1g, Protein 2g

Food Group Servings: 1 Serving = 1or more Vegetable, <1 dairy

Deviled Eggs

Stonyfield Farm provided this lighter recipe for stuffed eggs. A summer staple for backyard cookouts or elegant showers, these light and creamy eggs use yogurt in place of mayonnaise.

12 hard-boiled eggs
2 teaspoons mustard
1 teaspoon vinegar

2 teaspoons lemon juice
½ cup Stonyfield Farm low fat plain yogurt

1. Cut the peeled hardboiled eggs in half lengthwise and remove the yolks. Place yolks in a bowl and mash with a fork.
2. Add yogurt, mustard, vinegar and lemon juice. Mix well.
3. Season with salt and pepper to your taste.
4. Place filling in egg white halves and garnish with paprika.

Servings: 1. **Nutrition Facts**: Serving size: ¹⁄₁₂ of a recipe (2 halves), Amount Per Serving: Calories 95, Total Fat 6g, Saturated Fat 2g, Cholesterol 242mg, Sodium 87mg, Potassium 98mg, Total Carbohydrates 1.5g, Fiber .03g, Sugar 1g, Protein 7g

1 Serving = 1 Egg

Health Coach Tip:
♥ To reduce cholesterol you can toss out a couple of the egg yolks before mixing.

===

I adapted this recipe for a lower calorie, lower fat and 0 cholesterol deviled egg from Dr. Dean Ornish's *Everyday Cooking*. Try replacing the yolks with a mixture of made of garbanzo beans and spices. Mix the following in your food processor or blender, fill egg whites and top with paprika.

8 eggs, boiled and discard yolks
¼ cup chopped fresh parsley
½ teaspoon grated lemon zest or juice
⅛ teaspoon each salt and pepper
Paprika

One 15-ounce can garbanzo beans
3 teaspoons Dijon mustard
½ teaspoon garlic powder
2 tablespoon finely diced red onion

Nutrition facts: 2 deviled eggs. 35 calories, fat 0, cholesterol 0, protein 4g.

Garlic Bruschetta

When I visited the Garlic Festival in Gilroy, California, I returned with a new appreciation for the "Stinking Rose" as it has been known. For centuries, garlic has been thought to have many healing properties, and today new research has found that garlic helps stop plaque at early stages from keeping individual cholesterol particles from sticking to artery walls.

10 ripe roma tomatoes, chopped
2 Tablespoons fresh basil chopped
½ Romano cheese shredded
1 loaf French bread, unsliced

3 Tablespoons olive oil
4 garlic cloves, minced
Salt and pepper to taste

1. Slice French bread into 14 slices. Toast bread slices on both sides under broiler until golden.
2. Combine tomatoes, oil, basil, garlic, and cheese. Spread a spoonful of mixture on each bread slice and serve.

Servings: 14

Nutrition Facts: Serving size: ¼₁₄ of a recipe (4.2 ounces), Amount Per Serving: Calories 114, Total Fat 7.5g, Saturated Fat 3g, Cholesterol 16mg, Sodium 215mg, Potassium 250mg, Total Carbohydrates 6g, Fiber 1g, Sugar 2g, Protein 6g

Food Group Servings: 1 Serving = ½ Vegetable, 1 grains

Health Coach Tip:
- ♥ Garlic has been found to prevent blood clots, reduce blood pressure, and protect against infections.
- ♥ When combined with fresh lemon, lime or vinegar, garlic brings out the natural flavor in food, which means you need less salt.

Oven Fried Chicken Strips

Good homemade fried chicken is loved by many, though it is not low in calories or fat. You can enjoy this version of "fried" chicken strips without worry as an appetizer or for dinner with the appropriate portion size of mashed potatoes and carrot salad.

1 ½ cups buttermilk (or nonfat yogurt)　　2 tablespoons Dijon mustard
1 teaspoon sweet paprika　　　　　　　　¼ teaspoon cayenne pepper
¼ teaspoon garlic powder　　　　　　　　4 boneless skinless chicken breasts
¼ onion powder　　　　　　　　　　　　2 tablespoons buttery spread, melted
¼ teaspoon salt　　　　　　　　　　　　½ cup flour

1. Cut chicken into strips or leave whole and soak in buttermilk, at least 30 minutes before cooking.
2. Heat oven to 425 degrees. Melt butter in a 9 x 13 baking dish in the oven.
3. Stir together dry seasonings along with flour or biscuit mix in a pie plate. Coat chicken with mustard and dip in seasonings then place in baking dish with butter, flip over to coat both sides. Be careful, your baking dish will be hot.
4. Bake chicken breasts for 15 minutes, then turn over and bake for about 10 minutes more or until juice is no longer pink when thickest part is cut.

Servings: 8

Nutrition Facts: Serving size: ⅛ of a recipe (6.3 ounces), Amount Per Serving: Calories 206, Total Fat 5g, Saturated Fat 2, Cholesterol 78 mg, Sodium 231mg, Potassium 393mg, Total Carbohydrates 9g, Fiber <1g, Sugar 2g, Protein 30g

Food Group Servings: 1 Serving = 1.5 Meat 1 fat

Health Coach Tip:
♥ Parmesan Oven Fried Chicken Strips, decrease the flour to ⅓ cup, omit the salt and add ½ cup freshly grated parmesan cheese.

Potato Crisps with Ranch Dressing

Make your own ranch dressing and dip. This recipe is very fresh and lower in calories than traditional ranch in a bottle. Two ounces of this ranch dressing has only 22 calories and less than .5 grams of fat, as opposed to traditional ranch made with mayonnaise at 200 calories and 22 grams of fat for only two tablespoons. Keep in the refrigerator for a lighter fresh dressing on your salads and as a dip for fresh vegetables.

4 medium potatoes, unpeeled
1 tablespoon vegetable oil
½ cup light sour cream for dipping
1 clove garlic
2 pinches salt
¾ cup buttermilk, 1%

2 tablespoons lime juice
2 tablespoons parsley, chopped, divided
2 tablespoons chopped chives, divided
1 teaspoon garlic powder
1 teaspoon no salt seasoning

1. Preheat oven to 400 degrees.
2. Cut potatoes into ¼ inch slices, using a crinkle cutter if you have one. Place potatoes in a large bowl. Add oil and mix lightly. Add garlic powder, season salt, 1 each tablespoon chives and parsley and toss to coat evenly. Arrange potato slices in a single layer on a greased baking sheet. Do not overlap slices. Bake 40 to 45 minutes or until potatoes are browned and tender. Serve warm with light sour cream or ranch dressing.
3. For ranch dressing: mash together minced garlic and salt. Add to a small bowl together with buttermilk, lime juice, parsley, and chives until well blended. Taste and adjust seasoning with salt and pepper. Use immediately or refrigerate.

Servings: 8.

Nutrition Facts: Serving size: ⅛ of a recipe (4.6 ounces), Amount Per Serving: Calories 108, Total Fat 3g, Saturated Fat>1g, Cholesterol 4g, Sodium 278mg, Potassium 453mg, Total Carbohydrates 18g, Fiber 2g, Sugar 2g, Protein 3g

Food Group Serving: 1 Serving = 1 Vegetable, ½ Oils & fats

Health Coach Tip:
♥ Making this fresh recipe at home saves hundreds of calories, fat grams, undesirable preservatives and unhealthy oils used in restaurant dressings and fried foods.

Pumpkin Bread

Provided by Stonyfield Farm, this pumpkin bread is moist and delicious with just the right amount of sweetness thanks to the yogurt. Try it toasted.

3 eggs

1 cup sugar

⅓ cup vegetable oil

2 cups Stonyfield Organic Low Fat French Vanilla
  Yogurt or *any low-fat vanilla yogurt*

1 (16) ounce can pumpkin

2 teaspoons cinnamon

3 teaspoons nutmeg

1 ½ cups all-purpose flour

1 ½ cups whole wheat flour

1 teaspoon salt

1 tablespoon baking soda

½ tablespoon baking powder

1. Preheat oven to 400 degrees.
2. Grease and flour two 9 x 5 x 13 inch loaf pans.
3. Beat eggs until foamy, add sugar, oil, yogurt, pumpkin, cinnamon and nutmeg and mix well.
4. In a separate bowl sift together both flours, salt, baking soda and baking powder. Add dry ingredients slowly to the yogurt mixture and mix until moist.
5. Pour into both prepared loaf pans. Bake for 35-40 minutes. Loaves should be golden brown on top.
6. Cut each loaf into 12 slices.

Servings: 24

Nutrition Facts: Serving size: ¹⁄₂₄ of a recipe (2.7 ounces), Amount Per Serving: Calories 151, Total Fat 4., Saturated Fat >1g, Cholesterol 27.46mg, Sodium 356mg, Potassium 1141mg, Total Carbohydrates 25g, Fiber 1g, Sugar 12g, Protein 46g

Food Group Servings: 1 Serving = 1 Grains

Health Coach Tip: Add ½ cup chopped pecans or walnuts for added healthy fat and protein. Serve with sliced apples for a balanced snack.

Roasted Red Pepper Dip

Instead of using oil to marinate your vegetables before grilling, using this spicy alternative is a healthy option. Enjoy this colorful and healthy vegetable dip and marinade from Stonyfield. As a side, main dish or appetizer, or sandwiched with goat cheese inside some crusty bread, this robust sauce has a little kick.

1 cup Stonyfield or other plain fat-free yogurt *from cows fed without RBST or other hormones.*
1 (6) ounce jar roasted red peppers
4 cloves garlic
¼ teaspoon ground cumin
½ teaspoon sea salt

½ teaspoon ground pepper
¼ teaspoon crushed red pepper
1 eggplant
1 zucchini, cut off ends, slice lengthwise
1 summer squash, thinly sliced
1 onion, sliced into ½ inch thick rounds

1. Combine in food processor or blender the yogurt, red pepper, garlic, cumin, salt, pepper and crushed red pepper. Divide marinade and dip in half.
2. Arrange prepared vegetables on baking sheet, then coat with half of the marinade and refrigerate for one hour. Refrigerate the remaining marinade and dip.
3. Heat the grill to medium-high and coat with oil or cooking spray to prevent sticking. Grill vegetables for 2-3 minutes on each side. Serve with remaining dip.

Servings: 4

Nutrition Facts: Serving size: ¼ of a recipe (10.1 ounces), Amount Per Serving: Calories 100, Total Fat 1g, Saturated Fat <1g, Cholesterol 3.68mg, Sodium 223.83mg, Potassium 650.07mg, Total Carbohydrates 18g, Fiber 6g, Sugar 9g, Protein 6g

Food Group Servings: 1 Serving = 1 Vegetable

Spicy Popcorn

A fat free snack that will satisfy your taste buds.

12 cups pop corn popped
1 teaspoon dried oregano
¼ teaspoon garlic powder
Cooking spray

2 teaspoons paprika
½ teaspoon chili powder
¼ teaspoon ground cumin

1. Make herb and spice blend with paprika, oregano, chili powder, garlic powder and cumin. Mix well.
2. Make air popped or microwave popcorn.
3. Lightly spray with vegetable cooking spray.
4. Sprinkle popcorn with herb and spice blend, toss well and serve.

Servings: 6

Nutrition Facts: Serving size: ⅙ of a recipe (2 cups), Amount Per Serving: Calories 66, Total Fat <1g, Saturated Fat<1g, Cholesterol 0mg, Sodium 3.92mg, Potassium 80mg, Total Carbohydrates 13.g, Fiber 3g, Sugar .27g, Protein 2.26g

Food Group Servings

1 Serving = 1 Grains

Health Coach Tip:
♥ If you don't want your popcorn as spicy, change the spices to suit your taste. This is my husband's choice; I like mine with a garlic powder, a sprinkle of garlic salt, nutritional yeast flakes and parsley. It is very satisfying and saves you hundreds of calories, fat grams and hydrogenated oil from movie theatre popcorn.

Sweet & Salty Snack Mix

You can use any cereal you like for this snack mix, changing the combination depending on what you like. Aim to use a cereal with 3 or more grams of fiber. Bite size multi-grain bagel chips, pita chips or sesame snacks make a nice addition. Be careful to balance calories of the things you add. While this is a healthy snack providing fiber, protein and good fats, it can be high in calories if you eat more than a ½ cup serving.

2 cups Cheerios cereal
2 cups pretzels
½ cup walnuts, roughly chopped
½ cup raisins
1 teaspoon cinnamon

2 cups Wheat Chex cereal
½ cup almonds
¼ cup sunflower seeds
2 tablespoons Smart Balance margarine

1. Melt Smart Balance or Earth Balance Buttery Spread in a small bowl in microwave for a few seconds.
2. In a large bowl mix all the other ingredients.
3. Spread out on a large cookie sheet sprayed with cooking spray.
4. Preheat oven to 175 and bake for 1 hour, stirring every 15 minutes.
5. Store in an airtight container or pre-bag into ¼ cup servings.

Servings: 16

Nutrition Facts: **Serving size**: ¹⁄₁₆ of a recipe (½ cup), Amount Per Serving: Calories 217, Total Fat 7g, Saturated Fat >1g, Cholesterol 0mg, Sodium 470.73mg, Potassium 155mg, Total Carbohydrates 35g, Fiber 2g, Sugar 5g, Protein 5g

Food Group Servings: 1 Serving = 1 Grains, 1 nut/seed, 1 fats

Health Coach Tip:
♥ Resist buying pre-packaged snack mix, bagel chips, pretzels or any type of snack foods that has hydrogenated soybean oil or trans fats, *which are bad for your heart.*
♥ Look for individual foods with the least amount of ingredients possible to add to your own snack mix. You can use other cereals with a high fiber count (more than 3 grams).

Sweet Potato Spice Cake

Now you can have your cake and eat it too!

¾ cup whole wheat flour
¾ cup all purpose flour
½ cup sugar
1 teaspoon baking powder
½ teaspoon baking soda
1 large egg slightly beaten
2 cups crushed pineapple, in juice, drained

1 teaspoon cinnamon
½ teaspoon pumpkin pie spice
¼ cup raisins
1 cup mashed cooked sweet potatoes
½ cup fat-free milk
1 teaspoon vanilla extract
2 tablespoons brown sugar

1. Preheat oven to 350 degrees. Spray a 9 x 9 baking pan with cooking spray.
2. Sift together dry ingredients and stir in raisins.
3. Mix remaining ingredients together well, and then add to dry ingredients. Stir until moistened, but do not over mix.
4. Spread batter in pan. Bake 25 minutes or until toothpick comes out clean. Cool on rack.
5. When cooled, mix brown sugar with pineapple and top your snack cake. Cut into 9 pieces.

Servings: 9

Nutrition Facts: **Serving size**: ⅑ of a recipe (2.7 ounces), Amount Per Serving: Calories 210, Total Fat 7, Saturated Fat, <1g, Cholesterol 24mg, Sodium 147mg, Potassium 167mg, Total Carbohydrates 34g, Fiber 2g, Sugar 15g, Protein 4g

Food Group Serving: Serving = 1 Fruit, 1 grains, 1 fat

Health Coach Tip:
♥ You can substitute canned pumpkin to make this a pumpkin snack cake. Adding ½ cup chopped walnuts or pecans provides even more nutrition!

Darn Good Desserts

~

Better for You Banana Cream Pie

My version of "Banana Cream Pie" saves about 400 calories from my aunt's version, and mine is just a satisfying. Losing the crust will help you lose the pounds.

1 cup low fat vanilla yogurt
1 cup plain low fat yogurt

1 medium banana, peeled and sliced
8 Tablespoons canned light whipped topping

1. Mix yogurts together until creamy and spoon half equally into 4 small custard type cups.
2. Place sliced bananas on top of yogurt in cups.
3. Top with remaining yogurt and two tablespoons of canned light whipped cream on each one.

Servings: 4

Nutrition Facts: Serving size: ¼ of a recipe (6.6 ounces), Amount Per Serving: Calories 159, Total Fat 3g, Saturated Fat 2g, Cholesterol 11.3mg, Sodium 91.4mg, Potassium 497mg, Total Carbohydrates 27g, Fiber 1.5g, Sugar 20g, Protein 7g

1 Serving = ½ Fruit, ½ milk

Health Coach Tip:
♥ You can also break up a graham cracker in the bottom of the dishes before adding the yogurt to make a healthy crust to add a little crunch.

Chocolate Silken Tofu Pudding

Silken tofu has a smoother consistency and less bean taste than regular tofu. This is a great dessert for people who need a dairy free option. I use a protein powder made from whey. You can omit this.

2 tablespoons protein powder
1 tablespoon instant coffee
2 tablespoons cocoa powder, unsweetened
1 teaspoon vanilla

1 teaspoon cinnamon
¼ cup honey
12 ounces silken tofu

1. Place all ingredients into a blender and mix until smooth. Pour into individual dessert cups. Chill one hour.
2. Great served with sliced bananas or strawberries on top.

Servings: 4

Nutrition Facts: Serving size: ¼ of a recipe (4.5 ounces), Amount Per Serving: Calories 185, Total Fat 4g, Saturated Fat<1g, Cholesterol 0mg, Sodium 6.33mg, Potassium 257.33mg, Total Carbohydrates 236g, Fiber 3g, Sugar 23g, Protein 10g

1 Serving = 1 Beans/seed

Health Coach Tip:
♥ Tofu, while often made fun of by people who have not had it prepared properly, is high in calcium, iron, and protein, making it ideal for those who cannot have dairy products.

Cranberry Glazed Pears

Your family or guests will appreciate this fresh and different dessert.

2 cups cranberry juice, low calorie   6 pears
1 teaspoon cinnamon

1. In a saucepan, combine juice, and cinnamon. Bring to a boil over high heat. Meanwhile, peel pears, cut in half, and scoop out core. Put pears into the boiling juice mixture. Reduce heat to medium and simmer until pears are tender, about 15 minutes. Transfer pears and poaching liquid to a bowl and refrigerate at least 4 hours or overnight.
2. Remove pears. Put in individual serving dishes and spoon cranberry liquid over the pears. Serve with a dollop of vanilla yogurt.

Servings: 6

Nutrition Facts: Serving size: ⅙ of a recipe (11.9 ounces), Amount Per Serving: Calories 137, Total Fat <1g, Saturated Fat <1g, Cholesterol 0mg, Sodium 5mg, Potassium 270mg, Total Carbohydrates 36g, Fiber 7g, Sugar 24g, Protein <1g

Food Group Servings: 1 Serving = 1 fruit

Fudge Cake

I used to make a fudge sheet cake that used a pound of butter, two sticks in the cake, and two sticks of butter in the frosting. This one has a rich chocolate taste and is much lower in fat.

½ cup unsweetened cocoa
½ cup boiling water
2 cups sifted cake and pastry flour
1 teaspoon baking soda
½ teaspoon salt
1½ cups granulated sugar
⅓ cup Smart Balance margarine
2 teaspoons vanilla extract

2 large eggs
1 cup low fat buttermilk
1 ½ cups sifted powdered sugar
3 tablespoons unsweetened cocoa
2 tablespoons 1% low fat milk
1 teaspoon butter
½ teaspoon vanilla
2 tablespoons golden flax meal

1. Preheat oven to 350 degrees.
2. Coat a 13 x 9 inch baking pan with cooking spray.
3. To prepare sheet cake, combine ½ cup cocoa and water in a small bowl; cool.
4. Lightly spoon flour into dry measuring cup; level with a knife. Combine flour, baking soda, and salt, stirring well with a whisk. Place granulated sugar, Smart Balance, and 2 teaspoons vanilla in a large bowl; beat with a mixer at medium speed until well blended. Add eggs, one at a time, beating well after each addition. Beat in cocoa mixture. Add flour mixture, flax meal and buttermilk alternately to sugar mixture and beating well after each addition.
5. Pour batter into prepared pan and bake at 350 degrees or until the cake springs back when lightly touched. Cool in pan for 10 minutes on a wire rack.
6. For icing: combine the powdered sugar and 3 Tablespoons cocoa in a medium bowl, stirring well with a whisk. Add milk, butter, and ½ teaspoon vanilla; stir with a whisk until smooth. Spread icing over cake.

Servings: 12. **Nutrition Facts**: Serving size: ¹⁄₁₂ of a recipe (3.7 ounces), Amount Per Serving: Calories 251, Total Fat 5.g, Saturated Fat 2g, Cholesterol 37mg, Sodium 275mg, Potassium 149mg, Total Carbohydrates 47g, Fiber 2.g, Sugar 27g, Protein 5.g

Food Group Servings: 1 Serving = 1 Grains, 1 fats

Health Coach Tip:

- To keep your cake moist, be careful not to over bake and then frost it soon after it cools.
- Add flax meal because it is one of nature's richest plant source of Omega-3 fatty acids, an important part of our diet, but one that we are deficient in. Flax also provides additional fiber and phytoestrogens, and makes the cake moist by replacing saturated fat with a healthier fat. Desserts are extras. Eat from food groups through the day, stay active and have a treat when you have given your body the nutrition and exercise it needs.

Light & Easy Berry Trifle

Traditional trifles are made with heavy cream, sponge cake, and liqueur, which add a lot of calories and fat. To make this a little sweeter, you can spread the angel food cake with no sugar fruit jam before cutting it. Anyway you make this dessert, it will be a hit.

4 cups blueberries, sliced strawberries, raspberries, blackberries, or any mixture of berries desired.

2 cups plain, fat-free yogurt

2 cups low-fat vanilla yogurt

6 slices angel food cake

6 tablespoons canned whip cream

1. Use a large glass bowl or trifle bowl to display the bands of fruit.
2. Cut your angel food cake into cubes.
3. Mix together the yogurts.
4. Place a layer of the yogurt in the bottom of your bowl. Sprinkle with berries, making sure to also place them along the outside of the glass so they will show. Add a layer of diced angel cake.
5. Continue to layer the yogurt, berries and cake until you reach the top of the bowl, leaving a layer of berries for the top.
6. Just before you serve it, top with a few dollops of canned light whip cream.

Servings: 8

Nutrition Facts: Serving size: ⅛ of a recipe (7.7 ounces), Amount Per Serving: Calories 217, Fat 22, Total Fat 2.54g, Saturated Fat 1g, Cholesterol 8mg, Sodium 244mg, Potassium 37mg, Total Carbohydrates 42g, Fiber 2g, Sugar 25g, Protein 8.74g

Food Group Servings: 1 Serving = 1 Milk, 1 fruit, 1 grain, 1.2 fat

Health Coach Tips:
♥   This can be made for a brunch or dessert. In the summer, it is wonderful with fresh peaches and berries.
♥   Contrast the low calories and fat grams in this dessert to a national chain restaurant whose version of strawberry shortcake has 510 calories, 28 grams of fat, 80 mg of cholesterol and 44 grams of sugar.

Lower Calorie Mint Brownies

4 squares 1 ounce unsweetened baking chocolate

1½ cups sugar

½ cup egg substitute

¾ cup prune butter or apple butter

2 teaspoons vanilla extract

1½ cups unbleached all purpose flour

¼ teaspoon salt

¾ cup chopped walnuts or almonds (optional)

½ cup fat-free milk

Glaze:

1 cup confectioners' sugar

1 teaspoon vanilla extract

4 drops peppermint extract

5 teaspoons fat-free milk

1. Use a microwave or double boiler to melt the chocolate, being careful not to burn. If you do not have a double boiler, place a small saucepan into a larger one filled with water and cook over low heat, stirring constantly, until melted.
2. Place the chocolate in a large bowl, and stir in first the sugar, then the egg substitute, prune butter and vanilla extract. Stir to mix well. Stir in the flour, salt, and milk. Fold in walnuts.
3. Coat a 9 x 13 inch pan with nonstick cooking spray. Spread the batter evenly in the pan, and bake at 325 degrees for 35 to 40 minutes or until the center springs back to touch.
4. Be careful not to over bake. Cool to room temperature.
5. To make the GLAZE: Combine the glaze ingredients in a small bowl. If using a microwave oven, microwave the glaze uncovered at high power for 20 seconds or until runny. I like using a saucepan and cooking on the stovetop over medium heat for about a minute, stirring constantly.
6. Drizzle the glaze over the brownies and let harden before cutting into squares and serving. Use a ruler to mark before cutting into 30 squares of 5 by 6 rows.

Servings: 30. **Nutrition Facts**: Serving size: ⅟₃₀ of a recipe (1.9 ounces), Amount Per Serving: Calories 188, 11.g, Saturated Fat 6g, Cholesterol <1mg, Sodium 34mg, Potassium 197mg, Total Carbohydrates 24g, Fiber 3g, Sugar 14g, Protein 4g

1 Serving =2 Fats

Health Coach Tip:
♥ A great way to add extra fiber and moisten your brownies is to add a tablespoon or two of ground flax meal and or wheat germ to your batter. Delicious and nutritious. *Contrast the nutrition information in this brownie to a national chain restaurant with 470 calories per brownie, 18 fat grams, 80 mg cholesterol, and 57 grams of sugar.*

Luscious Low-fat Rocky Road "Ice Cream" Pie

1 crust cookie crust, chocolate
8 cups light ice cream, chocolate or
   rocky road
8 tablespoons nonfat chocolate syrup

6 tablespoons canned light whipped topping
½ cup miniature marshmallows
3 tablespoons chopped walnuts or almonds
   (optional)

1. Make this ice cream pie as soon as you return from the grocery store. The light ice cream will be just the right consistency to spoon into your cookie crust pie shell.
2. Drizzle the chocolate syrup all over the ice cream. Add the marshmallows and put into the freezer as soon as possible.
3. Let it set for at least 2 hours before serving. (Can be made a day ahead). Before serving take out of freezer and let sit for 10 minutes, then top with whipped topping and drizzle with a touch of chocolate syrup and chopped walnuts.

Servings: 8

Nutrition Facts: Serving size: ⅛ of a recipe (4 ounces), Amount Per Serving: Calories 220, Total Fat 8g, Saturated Fat 3g, Cholesterol 38mg, Sodium 113mg, Potassium 87mg, Total Carbohydrates 35g, Fiber <1g, Sugar 27g, Protein 5g

1 Serving = 1 Milk, 1 fats

Health Coach Tip:
♥ I know this isn't the most natural dessert. But the way I look at it, if you are going to have dessert once in a while, at least you can have one that has a lot less fat and calories than real ice cream, yet still tastes goods.
♥ Compare this 220 calorie serving to a national restaurant chain's version of mud pie which has 490 calories, 20 grams of fat and 52 grams of sugar, that's 13 teaspoons of sugar! This dessert has about 6-your daily allowance.

Marshmallow Nut Bars

Use brown rice crisp cereal. Nature's Path, Barbara's Bakery and others make an organic brown rice cereal.

4 cups miniature marshmallows
4 tablespoons buttery spread
6 cups crispy rice cereal
½ cup walnuts, finely chopped

½ cup walnuts, finely chopped
½ cup chopped pecans
½ cup golden raisins

1. Melt Smart Balance or Earth Balance in a large saucepan over low heat. Add marshmallows and stir constantly until completely melted. Remove from heat.
2. Add chopped nuts and raisins. Stir to blend. Add crisp rice cereal and stir until well coated. Using a buttered spatula, press into a 9 x 13 pan that has been sprayed with cooking spray. Cut into squares when cool.

Servings: 20

Nutrition Facts: Serving size: ⅟₂₀ of a recipe (1.1 ounces), Amount Per Serving: Calories 121, Total Fat 5g, Saturated Fat <1g, Cholesterol 0mg, Sodium 89mg, Potassium 62mg, Total Carbohydrates 19g, Fiber<1g, Sugar 9g, Protein 2g

Food Group Servings: 1 Serving = ½ Grains, <1 nut/seed, 1 fats

Health Coach Tip:
♥ Pre-wrap for individual lunch boxes treats or for an afternoon snack.

Pear Cranberry Crisp

If it isn't cranberry season, you can use blueberries, either way it is wonderful over fat-free vanilla frozen yogurt.

1 medium orange	½ teaspoon ground cinnamon
6 pears, peeled and thinly sliced	¼ cup packed brown sugar
1 cup fresh cranberries	¼ cup Smart Balance margarine
¾ cup granulated sugar	¾ cup rolled oats
5 tablespoons all purpose flour, divided	½ cup chopped pecans

1. Preheat oven to 350 degrees. Grate enough peel from orange to measure 1 teaspoon and squeeze enough juice to measure ¼ cup. In large bowl, combine orange juice, pears, cranberries, and granulated sugar. Add 2 Tablespoons of the flour and cinnamon and toss to coat. Place into a greased 8 or 9 inch square baking dish.
2. In a medium bowl, combine orange peel, the remaining 3 Tablespoons flour, and brown sugar. Using a knife and fork, cut in butter spread until mixture resembles coarse crumbs. Stir in pecans and oats. Sprinkle over fruit mixture. Bake 40 to 45 minutes or until golden brown.

Servings: 10

Nutrition Facts: Serving size: ¹⁄₁₀ of a recipe (6.9 ounces), Amount Per Serving: Calories 259, Total Fat 6.58g, Saturated Fat >1g, Cholesterol 0mg, Sodium 35.96mg, Potassium 250mg, Total Carbohydrates 51g, Fiber 6.g, Sugar 35g, Protein 2g

Food Group Servings: 1 Serving = 1 fruit, 1 nuts, 2 fats

Sour Cream Apple Pie

Once a high calorie pie made with piecrust, I created this version—without the crust and tastes even better without unnecessary fat. It is one of my favorite desserts.

2 cups chopped apples, diced with peels
3 tablespoons all purpose flour
½ cup sugar
Pinch of salt
½ cup low-fat sour cream *or fat-free plain yogurt*
1 egg beaten

1 teaspoon lemon juice
¼ cup Smart Balance Buttery Spread
½ cup brown sugar
½ cup all purpose flour
½ teaspoon cinnamon
1 teaspoon vanilla

1. Preheat oven to 425 degrees. Spray a pie plate with cooking spray.
2. Chop apples and set aside.
3. To make filling: Mix 3 Tablespoons flour with ½ cup sugar and pinch of salt in mixing bowl.
4. In another large mixing bowl combine sour cream, yogurt, egg, vanilla, and lemon juice.
5. Add dry ingredients a little at a time to wet ingredients while stirring. Stir in apples and mix well.
6. Pour apple mixture into prepared pie plate.
7. Make topping: Place ½ cup flour, ½ cup sugar, cinnamon and ¼ cup butter or Smart Balance margarine in a medium bowl, and cut with a knife and fork to mix, making pea size clumps.
8. Crumble mixture over top of pie, spreading evenly.
9. Bake at 425 degrees for 15 minutes, then reduce heat to 350 degrees and bake 30 minutes more.
10. Cool before serving and refrigerate leftover, if there are any.

Servings: 8. **Nutrition Facts: Serving size**: ⅛ of a recipe (3.5 ounces), Amount Per Serving: Calories 207, Total Fat 4g, Saturated Fat 1g, Cholesterol 30mg, Sodium 696mg, Potassium 121mg, Total Carbohydrates 40g, Fiber 1g, Sugar 29g, Protein 3g

Food Group Servings: 1 Serving = ½ Fruit, ½ milk 1 fat

Health Coach Tip:
- This recipe is so low in calories that you can afford to add ½ cup walnuts. This adds heart healthy fats and adds another dimension of flavor.
- You can reduce sugar by ¼ cup and it is still very good.

Tapioca Pudding

Tapioca is a classic comfort food. I use Bob's Red Mill all natural small pearl tapioca to make this creamy comforting dessert.

⅓ cup small pearl tapioca   ¾ cup water
2 ¼ cups 1% low fat milk   ¼ teaspoon salt
2 eggs, separated   ⅓ cup sugar
½ teaspoon vanilla

1. Soak small pearl tapioca in water for 30 minutes in a 1 ½ quart saucepan. Add milk, salt and lightly beaten egg yolks to tapioca and stir over medium heat until boiling.
2. Simmer uncovered over very low heat for 10 to 15 minutes. Stir often being careful not to burn.
3. Beat egg whites with sugar until soft peaks form. Fold about ¾ cup of hot tapioca into the egg whites, then gently fold mixture back into your saucepan.
4. Stir over low heat for about 3 minutes. Cool 15 minutes then add vanilla. Ladle 5 ounces into small individual serving cups and serve warm or chilled. Sprinkle with nutmeg or cinnamon.

Servings: 7

Nutrition Facts: Serving size: ⅐ of a recipe (4.8 ounces), Amount Per Serving: Calories 116, Total Fat 3g, Saturated Fat <1g, Cholesterol 64mg, Sodium 186mg, Potassium 140mg, Total Carbohydrates 20g, Fiber .07g, Sugar 14g, Protein 4g

Food Group Servings: 1 Serving = 1 milk

Health Coach Tip:
♥   To add fruit such as pineapple or blueberries, fold in before folding in the egg whites.

Grilled Peaches

This recipe is also delicious with glazed walnuts

4 peaches   8 tablespoons pecans, chopped
8 tablespoons blue cheese or feta

1. Wash and cut peaches in half, remove pits.
2. Place peach halves face down on a grill over medium heat. Grill for about five minutes, then turn over and grill for five minutes more, until the natural sugars begin to caramelize.
3. Remove peach halves from grill and fill cavities with 1 or 2 tablespoons of cheese.
4. Sprinkle with chopped pecans and drizzle with honey. Serve warm.

Servings: 8

Nutrition Facts: Serving size: ⅛ of a recipe (4ounces), Amount Per Serving: Calories 171, Total Fat 8g, Saturated Fat 1g, Cholesterol 5mg, Sodium 100mg, Potassium 208mg, Total Carbohydrates 25g, Fiber 2g, Sugar 24g, Protein 3g

Food group servings: 1 fruit, ½ dairy, 1 nuts

Peanut Butter Cocoa Protein Balls

This is a no bake dessert without any flour or sugar that will satisfy your sweet tooth.

1 cup peanut butter (*with no hydrogenated oil*)
½ cup raw oats
½ cup sunflower seeds
1 cup chopped walnuts or almonds
1 tablespoon water (*or more if necessary*)

⅓ cup cocoa powder, unsweetened
2 tablespoons protein powder
⅓ cup honey
2 teaspoons vanilla

1. Combine wet ingredients: honey, water, vanilla, peanut butter.
2. Chop sunflower seeds and walnuts until finely chopped.
3. Mix nuts and seeds with the rest of the dry ingredients. Then stir in peanut butter mixture.
4. Shape into balls about 1 tablespoon each in diameter and roll in coconut if desired.

Servings: 36

Nutrition Facts: Serving size: ⅟₃₆ of a recipe (.08 ounces), Amount Per Serving: Calories 110, Total Fat 8g, Saturated Fat 1g, Cholesterol 0mg, Sodium 42mg, Potassium 105mg, Total Carbohydrates 7g, Fiber 2g, Sugar 5g, Protein 4g

Food Group Servings: 1 nuts/seed, 1 fat

Health Coach Tip:
♥   Be sure to read the label before you choose your peanut butter. Avoid those with partially hydrogenated soybean oil.

Save Money and Calories Iced Mocha

Instead of spending money and gaining unwanted extra calories buying a coffee drink out, you will save money and calories by making your own delicious drink at home. Fat-free milk is a good choice to help you save fat grams. If you prefer, you may use almond milk, soy milk or other type of milk that is plain or low in sugar. Remember to read the label.

½ cup fat-free milk
½ cup coffee

1 cup crushed ice
2 tablespoons fat-free chocolate syrup

1. Mix in blender: crushed ice, fat-free milk or soy milk, coffee, and chocolate syrup or simply mix and pour into a tall glass over ice.

Servings: 1

Nutrition Facts: Serving size: 14.6 ounces, Amount Per Serving: Calories 134, Total Fat .056g, Saturated Fat <1g, Cholesterol 4mg, Sodium 184mg, Potassium 559mg, Total Carbohydrates 24g, Fiber 0g, Sugar 22g, Protein 8g

Food Group Servings: 1 Serving = ½ nuts, 1 milk

Health Coach Tip:
- Contrast the nutritional information with the blended drink from your local coffee house: Their 16 ounce drink, a blended mocha may have 410 calories, 15 grams of fat, 9 of saturated fat, 65 carbohydrates and 61 grams of sugar. *That's 15 teaspoons of sugar.*
- If you drink it in moderation, research suggests that coffee may offer protection against type 2 diabetes and other diseases. Coffee is rich in antioxidants, which help protect the vulnerable heart and blood vessels of a person with diabetes. However, coffee does have caffeine; one eight ounce cup of coffee can have between 90–200 mg, which can make you anxious and cause sleepless nights, so don't overdo. My version still contains 22 grams of sugar, or 4 teaspoons and should be considered a dessert. *Moderation is the key.*
- Be aware of artificial sweeteners, coffee creamers and syrups which are high in fat, sugar and artificial ingredients. Drinking these every day is an unhealthy habit.
- Milk, soy milk and almond milk have Vitamin D, B vitamins, calcium and other important nutrients which are good for bone health and are a naturally good way to add flavor to your coffee.

Printed in the United States
By Bookmasters